# Flesh and Bones of
# IMMUNOLOGY

Commissioning Editor: **Timothy Horne**
Development Editor: **Barbara Simmons**
Copy Editor: **Jane Ward**
Project Manager: **Frances Affleck**
Designer: **Jayne Jones**
Illustration Manager: **Mick Ruddy**

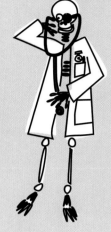

# Flesh and Bones of
# IMMUNOLOGY

## Matthew Helbert MBChB FRCP FRCPath PhD
Consultant Immunologist
Manchester Royal Infirmary
Manchester, UK

**Illustrations by** Robin Dean

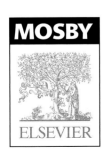

MOSBY

ELSEVIER

Edinburgh   London   New York   Oxford   Philadelphia   St Louis   Sydney   Toronto   2006

**MOSBY**

An imprint of Elsevier Limited

First published 2006

ISBN 0723433526

**British Library Cataloguing in Publication Data**
A catalogue record for this book is available from the British Library

**Library of Congress Cataloging in Publication Data**
A catalog record for this book is available from the Library of Congress

**Notice**
Neither the Publisher nor the Author assume any responsibility for any loss or injury and/or damage to persons or property arising out of or related to any use of the material contained in this book. It is the responsibility of the treating practitioner, relying on independent expertise and knowledge of the patient, to determine the best treatment and method of application for the patient.
*The Publisher*

Printed in Spain

The
Publisher's
policy is to use
**paper manufactured
from sustainable forests**

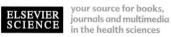

ELSEVIER
SCIENCE
your source for books,
journals and multimedia
in the health sciences

**www.elsevierhealth.com**

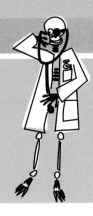

# Contents

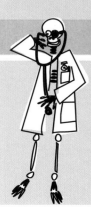

# Introduction: making sense of immunology

It is very important for students to have a good understanding of the immune system because so many diseases are caused by immunological problems. However, many students find Immunology a difficult topic and do not enjoy learning it. There are two main reasons for students struggling with immunology;

- some teachers get bogged down in the detail of how the immune system works, without providing an overview.
- some of the names of cells and molecules are very confusing.

In this book, the first section, The Big Picture, should be read first. This will give a simple overview of why we have an immune system and how the different components fit together. Take your time to read this section and make sure you really understand the material. This knowledge can then be used as a map to help you through the more detailed information that follows. Section 2 contains 50 'high-return' facts that are the vital 'bare bones' on which immunology is based. Section 3 'fleshes out' each of these facts.

## Names of molecules

Over the past 100 years, several thousand different immune system molecules and cells have been discovered. Fortunately, you only need to know about 100 of these. To help you follow the many abbreviations, a list is given at the end of this introduction. At the end of the book, a short glossary will give succinct descriptions of the major components. The discovery of the immune molecules took place in a haphazard fashion and so their nomenclature often lacks a coherent logic. For the first 70 years it was not at all clear how all the different cells and molecules fitted together. So some of the components have very strange names. For example Toll-like receptors are human molecules named after a molecule found in flies, called 'Toll'!

Other molecules have strange abbreviations, for example the CD (cluster of differentiation, for example CD4) and the IL (interleukin, for example IL-1) molecules. These molecules were given these abbreviations in the order they were discovered. Which means that the numbers do not very often relate to the function of the molecules.

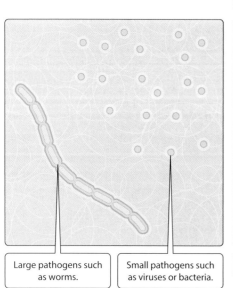

Large pathogens such as worms.

Small pathogens such as viruses or bacteria.

Cells of the innate immune system

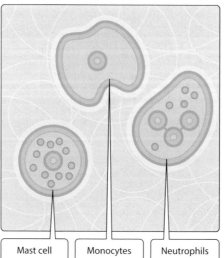

Mast cell | Monocytes | Neutrophils

Lymphocytes are the cells of the adaptive immune system

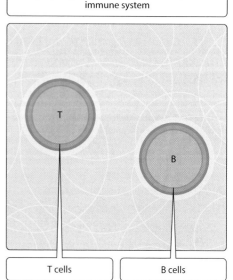

T cells | B cells

**Intro. Fig 1**

Although cells of the immune system are present in many tissues, they are also usually found as white cells (or leukocytes) in the blood. The leukocytes can be divided into two types. Myeloid cells are only produced in the bone marrow and include neutrophils, macrophages, eosinophils and mast cells. These cells belong to the innate immune system; all innate immune system components are coloured green in this book. The other type of leukocytes is the lymphocytes. These are further divided into B cells and T cells and form the adaptive immune system (coloured blue) (Intro. Fig. 1).

When a cell has a molecule on its surface, immunologists say that a cell expresses the molecule. Many of the molecules are involved in communication between these different populations (Intro. Fig. 2). There are two main types of molecules:

- *ligands* are pairs of molecules that form bridges directly between cells
- *receptors* are molecules that can bind on to soluble messenger molecules called cytokines.

Cytokines were originally referred to as interleukins, generally abbreviated to IL. Not all intercellular messenger molecules follow this nomenclature though, and in the text you will learn about other cytokines, such as interferons (IFN), tumour necrosis factor (TNF) and granulocyte-macophage colony-stimulating factor (GM-CSF). Cells can also express a different type of receptor that is able to recognize microorganisms.

The whole purpose of the immune system is to deal with microorganisms. In this book they are coloured yellow. Remember that there are many different types of microorganism and the final part of this book explains how the immune system deals with all of these. Unfortunately, the immune system does not always work well and can sometimes cause disease. You will read all about this in the later parts.

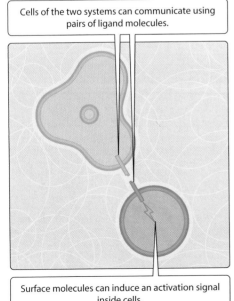

Cells of the two systems can communicate using pairs of ligand molecules.

Surface molecules can induce an activation signal inside cells.

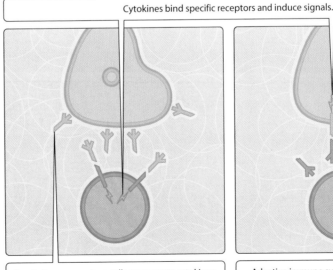

Cytokines bind specific receptors and induce signals.

Innate immune system cells can secrete cytokines.

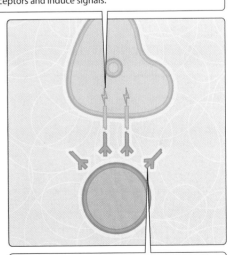

Adaptive immune system cells can also secrete cytokines.

**Intro. Fig 2**

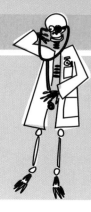

# Abbreviations used in this book

| | |
|---|---|
| AIDS | acquired immunodeficiency disease |
| CRP | C-reactive protein |
| CVID | common variable immunodeficiency |
| G-CSF | granulocyte-macrophage colony-stimulating factory |
| HIV | human immunodeficiency virus |
| HLA | human leukocyte antigen |
| ICAM | intercellular adhesion molecule |
| IFN | interferon |
| IL | interleukin |
| MBL | mannose-binding lectin |
| MHC | major histocompatibility complex |
| SCID | severe combined immunodeficiency |
| SLE | systemic lupus erythematosus |
| Th | T helper |
| TLR | Toll-like receptor |
| TNF | tumour necrosis factor |

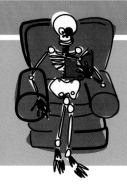

# The big picture

*The key to understanding immunology is to consider it as a whole. The immune system is made up of several hundred interacting genes, molecules and cells (you only need to know about 50 or so of these). When looking at the individual components, always try to put them in the context of the big picture. You don't need to remember everything you read in this section. Just try to understand how the components fit together.*

The immune system has one fundamental task—to prevent the body from being taken over by infection. When you consider the range of pathogens that threaten the body, you start to become aware of the scale of this task. Viruses, because of their simple genomes, are pathogens that are only able to survive inside host cells. At the other end of the scale, there are worms that live inside body cavities and can grow up to hundreds of centimetres in size. In between these two extremes are the bacteria, fungi, and protozoans. Different immune mechanisms are required to fend off different types of pathogen.

Pathogens and their hosts have evolved side by side (Fig. 1.1). Early in evolutionary terms, pathogens were unsophisticated and easily fended off by immune systems far more simplistic than those of today. With time, pathogens developed specialist strategies for overcoming the host immune system. This led to pressure for increasing complexity in the host defences. Around the time that vertebrates began to evolve, there was a 'big bang'

revolution in the immune system, and, as a result of this, an adaptive immune system developed.

The human immune system is made up of two major branches:

- innate immunity
- adaptive immunity.

## INNATE IMMUNITY

The innate immune system provides the body's first line of defence against pathogens. The most important basic defence of the innate immune system is a thick impervious **skin**, providing a barrier. Internal body surfaces have to be much thinner in order to absorb nutrients and oxygen and for excretory products to diffuse out. These surfaces are protected by more specialized means, for example a layer of mucus in the respiratory tract with cilia that waft pathogens out of the body. These basic defences are prone to damage, for example by injury; when this happens, pathogens such as bacteria and fungi can enter the body.

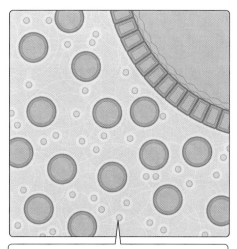

The most primitive pathogens live in the extracellular space, e.g. most bacteria and fungi.

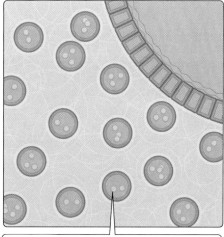

Other pathogens are hidden inside cells, including some bacteria, fungi, protozoans and all viruses.

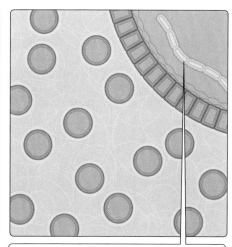

Larger pathogens live on mucosal surfaces, for example worms.

**Fig. 1.1** Pathogens and host have evolved side by side.

**Phagocytes** have evolved to be an early means of defending against invading organisms. They are free-living cells capable of moving throughout the body and engulfing pathogens. There are two types of phagocyte: **neutrophils** and **macrophages**. They express a handful of specialized receptors that can recognize molecules present on the surface of invading pathogens. These receptors are sometimes called **pattern recognition molecules**. They recognize repeated sugar molecules on the surface of pathogens. If the receptors bind onto pathogens, they are phagocytosed and held in an intracellular vacuole. Phagocytes then release proteolytic enzymes, which usually destroy the pathogen. Phagocytes also release proteins (known as chemokines) into the extracellular space, and these attract more phagocytes to the site of infection (Fig. 1.2). Consider what happens when you get a splinter in your finger. The collection of pus that forms 24 hours after the injury is a mixture of dead neutrophils and bacteria.

For pathogens that are too big to be phagocytosed, other specialized cells dump enzymes onto the surface of the pathogen. **Mast cells** are an example of these degranulating cells.

The risks of infection are so great that often the immune system evolves two ways of dealing with the same problem. The **complement** system evolved in parallel with phagocytes and is an even more rapid way of dealing with infections. Complement is a cascade of serum enzymes that is activated by sugars on the surface of pathogens. This can happen because pattern recognition molecules are able to distinguish between host and pathogen sugars. Activation of a single complement molecule

makes it enzymatically active and so it can activate more molecules, in a fashion reminiscent of the clotting cascade. There are several results of complement activation, the most potent being the **membrane attack complex**, which can punch holes in pathogens. Activation of complement also increases phagocytosis by attracting more phagocytes to the site of infection and by making pathogens more attractive targets for phagocytosis (Fig. 1.2).

The combination of the phagocyte and the complement systems is effective in dealing with pathogens living outside cells: most bacteria and fungi. An obvious place for pathogens to hide is inside cells, where complement and phagocytes cannot reach them. Some bacteria and fungi can do this, but the main group of pathogens that has evolved to live intracellularly is the viruses. The intracellular pathogens, especially viruses, successfully evaded the phagocytes and complement of the evolving immune system, and a new response had to develop in order to fight back. In response to intracellular infections, many cells throughout the body secrete **interferons**. These are proteins that are able to switch off the cellular machinery necessary for viral replication and they are reasonably good at combating viral infections (Fig. 1.3).

The early immune system thus consisted of barriers, phagocytes, complement and interferons. It was good at dealing with extracellular bacteria and fungi and reasonably good at dealing with intracellular viruses. A problem with this early, innate immune system was that each time the host was exposed to pathogens, the response had to start from zero: the host could be infected with same pathogen again and again.

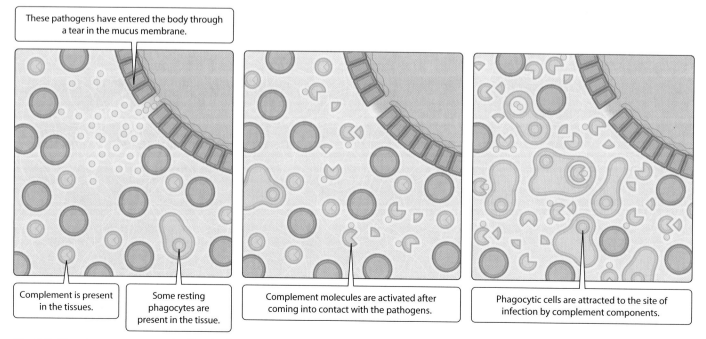

These pathogens have entered the body through a tear in the mucus membrane.

Complement is present in the tissues.

Some resting phagocytes are present in the tissue.

Complement molecules are activated after coming into contact with the pathogens.

Phagocytic cells are attracted to the site of infection by complement components.

**Fig. 1.2** The phagocyte system is effective but rather slow.

## ADAPTIVE IMMUNITY

The adaptive immune system evolved at about the same time as early vertebrates. Vertebrates tend to live longer than invertebrates and face a lifelong risk of infection, especially by intracellular viruses. The larger size of vertebrates meant, for the first time, that organisms were prey to parasitic worms living in body cavities. Several adaptations had to take place before new receptor molecules could be used to detect the newer intracellular pathogens and large worms that had evolved to live inside body cavities.

The older innate system used a handful of receptors to bind with pathogens, each of which was coded for by a unique gene. A key feature of the adaptive immune system was that it dramatically increased the number of receptors for any possible pathogen molecule. To have a single gene for each of these unique receptors would take up far too much room on the genome. Cells of the adaptive immune system use a unique system to overcome this lack of space. To increase the number of potential receptors, cells of the adaptive immune system randomly cut and paste segments from a pool of genes. By doing so, these cells are able to express billions (up to $10^{18}$) of new receptor molecules. These receptors, generated through genetic recombination, are expressed on specialized lymphocytes called **T** or **B cells**. The generation of this immense diversity is a key feature of the adaptive immune system.

### T cells

The newly evolved T cell receptors are expressed on the surface of T cells and are only able to recognize intracellular infections if pathogen-derived molecules are present on the surface of the infected cell. A mechanism had to evolve to enable a cell to sample the complete range of proteins inside its body and display these on its surface. To do this, small quantities of intracellular proteins are lysed into small fragment peptides, which are then pumped into the endoplasmic reticulum. These peptides give a representative profile of all the peptides inside the cell, including any belonging to intracellular pathogens. For this system to work, the peptides from any given cell have to be firmly bound to the cell surface. Vertebrate cells express a family of molecules, known as **MHC** molecules, that are able to bind small peptides derived from the intracellular protein pool and display them on the cell surface. The human MHC is known as the **HLA** (human leukocyte antigens). There are different classes of MHC with varying function. Class I molecules display peptides from intracellular proteins, including those of pathogens. They have a small groove and the peptides lie bound inside this. Some T cells use their recombinant receptors to distinguish between host peptides and any abnormal pathogen peptides, usually from viruses. If they detect abnormal pathogen peptides, these T cells can either try to inhibit viral replication by secreting interferon or actually kill the cell and its contents. These cells are called **cytotoxic T lymphocytes** (Fig. 1.4).

This system is also used effectively to detect extracellular pathogens. If a cell takes up any extracellular pathogen, or fragment of pathogen, these can be degraded into peptides inside a phagocytic lysosome. These peptides bind to another specialized surface molecule, called **MHC class II**. The T cells that recognize these peptides derived from the extracellular environment are called **helper T cells** (Th cells). On recognizing the presence of pathogen peptides, these cells help other parts of the immune system combat the infection.

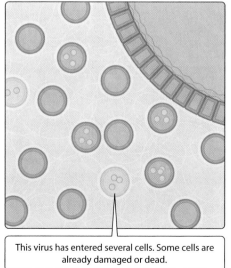
This virus has entered several cells. Some cells are already damaged or dead.

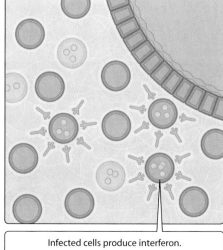
Infected cells produce interferon.

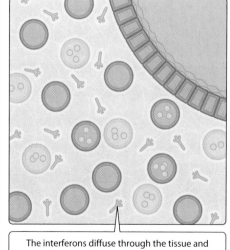
The interferons diffuse through the tissue and prevent some cells becoming infected. There is already considerable damage at this point.

**Fig. 1.3** Interferons are secreted to combat intracellular pathogens.

The pathogen-derived peptides recognized by the two types of T cell are called **antigens**. Antigens recognized by T cells are only a few amino acid residues long. They have to be quite small to fit inside the groove on the MHC molecules. Any given T cell receptor can only recognize one specific amino acid sequence forming one peptide.

Because the recombination process that is used to generate T cell receptors happens at random, there is always a risk that a T cell may happen to recognize a peptide derived from normal host proteins, rather than from a pathogen. This could result in T cells attacking normal host cells. To prevent this from happening, T cells that recognize host antigens are killed before they ever reach the circulation. This happens in the thymus.

To sum up.

■ T cells express one of several billion T cell receptors, which recognize peptides bound to the groove of MHC molecules.

■ These receptors are generated through genetic recombination.

■ T cells that could recognize harmless host (self) peptides are deleted in the thymus.

■ T cells that respond to peptides derived from intracellular pathogens are called cytotoxic T cells.

■ T cells that respond to peptides from extracellular sources are called helper T cells.

Several billion T cell receptors potentially exist. This would enable the immune system to recognize an almost unlimited range of pathogen peptides. In fact the range of peptides recognized by T cells is more limited by the groove on the MHC molecule. Any given MHC molecule can only bind a few hundred different peptides.

Nature has developed an interesting way of overcoming this constraint. Every individual inherits slightly different genes for the MHC molecules. This means that any two random individuals have MHC molecules that bind different pathogen-derived peptides. If a pathogen attacked a population, the constraints applied by MHC may mean that some individuals would not bind important peptides and could not respond to the infection. Other individuals, with different MHC molecules, would respond well. So even though the MHC applies a constraint to the diversity of an individual's immune system, at a population level, the mixture of different types of MHC molecule means that some individuals will always survive. You need to know a little about the genetic differences in MHC because it is this molecule that causes rejection reactions when organs are transplanted between people with different MHC molecules.

Pathogens will inevitably evolve ways of overcoming the immune system. Some viruses (the herpesvirus family) have specialized in this. When these viruses infect cells, they prevent the expression of MHC molecules. Without MHC to bind virus antigens, T cells have no way of recognizing that infection is taking place.

The host immune system has, in turn, overcome this trick. **Natural killer cells** are a special type of lymphocyte that has receptors for MHC. If MHC is absent, they will kill the cell and any virus it contains.

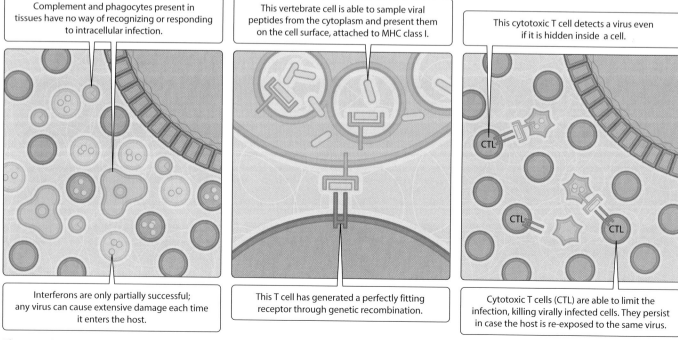

Complement and phagocytes present in tissues have no way of recognizing or responding to intracellular infection.

This vertebrate cell is able to sample viral peptides from the cytoplasm and present them on the cell surface, attached to MHC class I.

This cytotoxic T cell detects a virus even if it is hidden inside a cell.

Interferons are only partially successful; any virus can cause extensive damage each time it enters the host.

This T cell has generated a perfectly fitting receptor through genetic recombination.

Cytotoxic T cells (CTL) are able to limit the infection, killing virally infected cells. They persist in case the host is re-exposed to the same virus.

**Fig. 1.4** Cytotoxic T lymphocytes can kill cells containing pathogens.

## B cells and immunoglobulins

B cells are a type of lymphocyte and, like T cells, they produce receptors through genetic recombination. Unlike T cells, not all the B cell receptors stay on the surface of the B cell. Some of these receptors are actively secreted into the intercellular space and into body cavities. The free B cell receptor molecules are known as immunoglobulin (Ig) or antibody. Another difference from the T cell receptor is that immunoglobulins do not need to bind antigen lying in the groove of MHC. Immunoglobulin can bind soluble antigens or antigens on the surface of pathogens (Fig. 1.5). There are several different types of immunoglobulin molecule, called IgM, IgG, IgA and IgE. Any given B cell will secrete one type.

Each class of immunoglobulin has a specialized role. **IgM** stays in the blood and intercellular fluid and binds onto the surface of pathogens. It then activates components of the innate immune system. It stimulates complement and phagocytosis.

The IgA and IgG classes are only found in mammals. IgG is present in most body compartments and is able to activate phagocytosis. IgA is actively secreted across mucosal surfaces and so protects the gut and respiratory tract.

Newborn animals are very prone to infection because of the immaturity of their immune systems. In mammals, immunoglobulins play a very special role. IgG is actively pumped across the placenta and breast milk contains IgA. These protect young mammals from infection. This means that mammals need to have fewer offspring.

One type of immunoglobulin, IgE, evolved to combat worm infections. The IgE defence system requires interaction with mast cells in the mucosa (host) underlying the worms. IgE produced by B cells binds to the surface of mast cells. If the bound IgE recognizes worm antigen, it cause the mast cell to release chemicals which make the gut produce increased amounts of mucus and contract (Fig. 1.5). The worm loses its grip on the gut lining and is expelled during the gut contraction.

Apart from the ability to create diverse T and B receptors, the other key feature of the adaptive immune system is *memory*. When the adaptive immune system first encounters a pathogen, there may be very few T or B cells with receptors that are capable of recognition. During the immune response, T and B cells that recognize the pathogen divide rapidly, producing many more daughter cells, each with appropriate receptors. Many of these cells will survive for many years after the infection has been combated. These cells, which are still increased in number, will be able to respond to pathogen should it be encountered again. This is the basis of immunological memory.

By transferring immunoglobulins to the newborn, there is actually a temporary transfer of the mother's immunological memory.

Vaccines have saved many millions of lives around the world and they are also an example of immunological memory that you need to understand. In this case, harmless purified pathogen antigen is administered and it is this that triggers the development of memory.

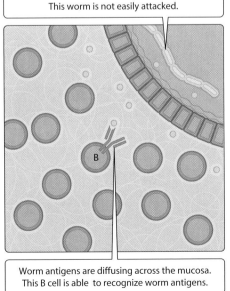

This worm is not easily attacked.

Worm antigens are diffusing across the mucosa. This B cell is able to recognize worm antigens.

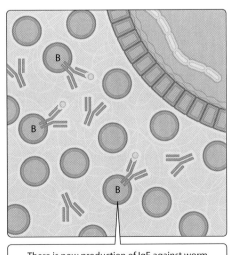

There is now production of IgE against worm antigen by B cells.

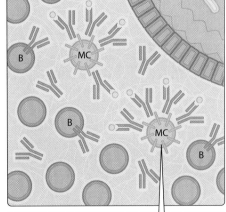

IgE bound to most cells is cross-linked. The mast cells release substances that cause the gut to contract.

**Fig. 1.5** B cells produce immunoglobulins (antibodies).

### ■ THE IMMUNE SYSTEM: A NETWORK

By now you should understand why the immune system has different components, each adapted to combat specific types of infection. The seven key components are shown in Table 1.1. None of these components work alone. For example, phagocytes of the innate immune system are able to present antigen on their MHC molecules to the T cells of the adaptive system. Immunoglobulin molecules of the adaptive system are able to facilitate the effects of complement and phagocytes.

T helper cells have a coordinating role in the immune system. They 'decide' whether or not the immune system is dealing with extracellular pathogens (in which case immunoglobulin production is paramount) or intracellular infections (in which case cytotoxic T lymphocytes are required) (Fig. 1.6).

**Table 1.1** COMPONENTS OF THE IMMUNE SYSTEM.

|  | **Innate** | **Adaptive** |
|---|---|---|
| Adapted for extracellular organisms | Phagocytes, complement | Immunoglobulin |
| Coordinating role |  | T helper cells |
| Adapted for intracellular organisms | Interferon | Cytotoxic T cells, natural killer cells |

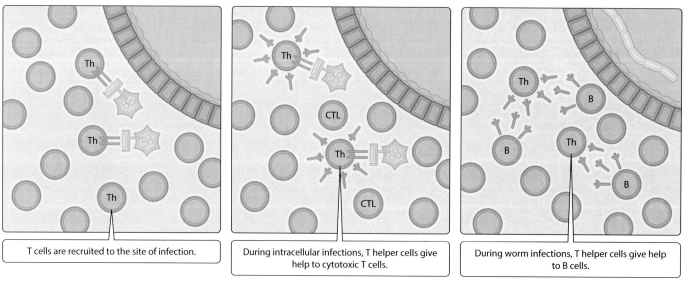

T cells are recruited to the site of infection.

During intracellular infections, T helper cells give help to cytotoxic T cells.

During worm infections, T helper cells give help to B cells.

**Fig. 1.6** T helper cells direct the adaptive immune system to produce the most appropriate response to infection.

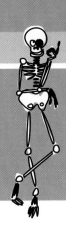

# High-return facts

*This section lays out the major underlying principles. High-return facts are the core concepts, the underlying principles of immunology. They help to focus learning and provide an overview to build knowledge around. They are the bare bones on which the subject hangs. Learning these high-yield facts guards against major gaps in knowledge.*

## ■ GENERAL PRINCIPLES

**1** The immune system has two parts: the innate and adaptive system. The innate system is either present all the time or activated very quickly. It responds in exactly the same way to any pathogen. Anatomical barriers are part of the innate immune system and consist of the skin, the low pH found in the stomach, and the cilia and mucus of the respiratory tract.

**2** The innate immune system uses about a dozen pattern recognition molecules to recognize that infection is taking place. These are present in solution or on the surface of innate immune system cells. Pattern recognition molecules recognize substances (for example double-stranded RNA and certain sugars) that are not present in normal mammalian cells.

**3** Complement is a family of serum protein circulating in an inactive pro-enzyme form. Complement can be activated by sugars present on the surface of pathogens. Activation of complement results in damage to the pathogen.

**4** Phagocytes include neutrophils and macrophages and are cellular components of the innate immune system. These cells have receptors for extracellular pathogens, such as many bacteria. When phagocytes encounter pathogens, they ingest them, forming a phagosome. The phagocytosed pathogen is killed by the respiratory burst, proteolytic enzymes and defensins.

**5** Cytokines are chemical mediators produced by cells of the innate and adaptive immune system responding to infection. One of the roles of cytokines is to switch on the acute-phase response, consisting of fever and changes in plasma proteins. C-reactive protein (CRP) is a plasma protein produced at increased levels during an acute-phase response. The most exaggerated form of acute-phase reaction is septic shock.

**6** Degranulating cells include mast cells and eosinophils. They are adapted to deal with pathogens, such as worms, that are too large to be phagocytosed. On exposure to pathogens, granules contained in these cells are released onto the surface of the worm. These cells also use metabolites of arachidonic acid to help to clear the worm infection.

**7** The interferons are a family of chemical mediators released by virus-infected cells. Interferons switch off viral replication inside cells. Interferons have been used to treat some chronic infections. Interferons are examples of 'danger signals', which the innate immune system uses to alert the adaptive immune system that infection is taking place.

**8** The adaptive immune response differs from the innate system in that it recognizes specific antigen. Antigen is recognized by immunoglobulin or T cells. T cells recognize peptide antigens from intracellular or phagocytosed pathogens that have been processed and displayed on HLA (MHC) molecules.

**9** T cells express receptors that recognize peptide antigen lying in the groove of HLA molecules. The T cell receptors have variable domains that recognize the antigenic peptide. Genetic recombination is used to create genes for millions of different T cell receptors.

**10** T cell precursors randomly splice together gene segments to produce a unique gene for a receptor molecule. There are a number of different segments available for this process. Random errors at the site of gene segment joining add further diversity to the T cell receptor genes.

**11** Different subsets of T cells express the surface molecules CD4 or CD8. When the T cell receptor recognizes antigen plus HLA, signals are transmitted through the cytoplasm to the nucleus. These signals are initiated when CD3, the T cell receptor and CD4 or CD8 form an immunological synapse. The cytoplasmic tails of these molecules then activate kinases.

**12** In the thymus, only T cells that recognize self-HLA survive a first wave of positive selection; T cells that are activated by subsequent exposure to normal self-antigen are destroyed through a process called negative selection. In this way, T cells become self-restricted, but tolerant to self-antigen.

**13** The genes for the HLA molecules differ from person to person: they are polymorphic. The protein produced by each HLA allele is only able to bind a few different peptide antigens. This has evolved to limit the spread of infection through a population, but it also has implications for transplantation.

**14** The two main types of T cell population are cytotoxic T cells (CTL) and T helper (Th) cells. Cytotoxic T cells recognize and attack other cells containing intracellular pathogens, such as viruses. Cytotoxic T cells express the CD8 membrane molecule and only recognize antigen associated with HLA class I molecules. Natural killer cells are specialized cells that kill cells when HLA is absent. Both natural killer and cytotoxic T cells kill by inducing apoptosis.

**15** The adaptive immune system uses antibody to recognize macromolecular antigen. Macromolecules can be made up of protein, sugars, lipids or nucleic acids. Macromolecules produced by pathogens do not require antigen processing.

**16** Antibody has two separate immunoglobulin chains— the light chain and the heavy chain—and these are used to recognize antigen: B cells produce immunoglobulin chains using similar genetic recombination events.

**17** The different classes of immunoglobulin (IgM, IgG, IgA, IgE and IgD) are produced by switching the constant region gene segments of the heavy chain. IgM is produced first by any B cell. Each immunoglobulin class has a distinct functional role.

**18** B lymphocytes are produced in the bone marrow. They have membrane-bound antibodies as their cell surface receptors and are prone to negative selection, so that only self-tolerant B cells leave the bone marrow. Most B cells require T cell help in the periphery, also to ensure B cells are tolerant to self-antigen.

**19** B cells initially produce IgM but switch to production of other immunoglobulin classes after interaction with T cells. After class switching, B cells undergo somatic hypermutation in order to produce antibody of highest affinity.

**20** Primed B cells that have undergone class switching can produce either plasma cells (which produce large amounts of immunoglobulin) or memory B cells. A very different type of B cell is the T-independent B cell, which responds to bacterial sugars without undergoing recombination.

**21** Naïve T cells are activated by antigen and dendritic cells to become memory T helper cells. Memory T helper cells are able to respond to antigen quickly, migrate to many sites in the body and have a coordinating role in the immune system. Th1 cells promote the activity of cytotoxic T cells, while Th2 cells promote antibody production by B cells.

**22** The components of the adaptive immune system exist in specific sites; the primary lymphoid organs (bone marrow, thymus) provide specific environments for the maturation of lymphocytes. The secondary lymphoid organs are sites where antigen is trapped and comes into contact with lymphocytes. The lymph nodes, spleen and mucosa-associated lymphoid tissue (MALT) are all secondary lymphoid organs.

**23** During infection, neutrophils adhere to the vascular endothelium (margination). Then, they move through the endothelial wall via diapedesis. This is achieved through binding of specific ligand pairs on neutrophils and endothelium, including selectins and addressins. Similar ligand pairs control lymphocyte trafficking; naïve cells migrate to the lymph node cortex while memory T cells migrate to specific tissues.

**24** The innate immune system can clear acute bacterial infection, although antibody makes this process more effective. Acute inflammation and the production of pus is part of this process. Antibody can also prevent future acute bacterial infections.

**25** The innate immune system cannot effectively clear acute viral infection; Th1 responses are required for sterilizing immunity. Antibody cannot eradicate established infection but can prevent reinfection with exactly the same virus.

**26** Chronic infection occurs when the immune system cannot clear infection, for example tuberculosis. Specialized Th1 responses are able to control most cases of tuberculosis, and granuloma may be produced, requiring IL-12 from macrophages and interferon-γ from Th1 cells.

## HYPERSENSITIVITY

**27** Inflammation is a normal response to infection. In some situations, the immune response causes more damage than the pathogen; this is a type of hypersensitivity. Hypersensitivity can also take place when the immune system responds to harmless substances from the environment or even normal body components (autoimmune disease). Hypersensitivity is classified into four different types with different mechanisms and timings.

**28** Type 1 hypersensitivity reactions take place immediately after exposure to antigen and cause allergic reactions. Th2 cells drive IgE production. IgE binds to mast cells, which degranulate on exposure to antigen. These reactions are more common in individuals with genetic predisposition (atopy) who have been bought up in hygienic conditions.

**29** Examples of allergic reactions include angio-oedema, anaphylaxis, urticaria, atopic eczema, rhinitis and asthma. The symptoms of allergy depend on the which organs are exposed to the allergen.

**30** Type 2 hypersensitivity is antibody-mediated cytotoxic hypersensitivity. Antibodies are directed against cell surface antigens, causing cell destruction. This most commonly occurs in blood transfusion reactions and haemolytic disease of the newborn.

**31** Type 3 is immune-complex-mediated hypersensitivity. Antigen–antibody complexes are deposited in tissues and activate the complement pathways, leading to an inflammatory response. The immune complexes can trigger a local reaction, for example humidifier lung, or circulate and cause disease in the kidneys, joints and skin.

**32** Type 4 is cell-mediated hypersensitivity. It is a delayed reaction and is mediated through Th1 cells. Some type 4 reactions take place in response to pathogens, for example in tuberculosis; harmless environmental antigens are involved in contact dermatitis. Tumour necrosis factor appears to be a key cytokine in mediating the pathology of delayed hypersensitivity.

## AUTOIMMUNITY

**33** Some autoimmunity is normal and is detectable in healthy people. More severe autoimmunity develops when there is a failure of self-tolerance, so T and B cells are able to respond to normal body antigens. Tolerance can break down because of failure of negative selection in the thymus: this usually has a genetic basis. Tolerance can also break down in the peripheral tissues, most often because of environmental factors such as infection.

**34** Tolerance breakdown results in hypersensitivity reactions, leading to autoimmune disease. In some diseases, autoantibodies attack healthy tissues, using type 2 hypersensitivity mechanisms. These diseases include autoimmune haemolytic anaemia, Hashimoto's thyroiditis, Grave's disease and pernicious anaemia. Autoantibodies are used to help to diagnose these diseases.

**35** Circulating immune complexes (type 3 hypersensitivity) can also cause autoimmune disease. One of the best examples is systemic lupus erythematosus (SLE). Tests for specific autoantibodies are used to diagnose SLE.

**36** Rheumatoid arthritis is a very common autoimmune disease caused by delayed (type 4) hypersensitivity. Treatment is improving as we understand more about how the hypersensitivity reactions trigger disease.

## MALIGNANCY

**37** Cells of lymphocyte origin can sometimes become malignant. This can occur as a result of translocation of an oncogene to an immunoglobulin promoter. In other cases the Epstein–Barr virus is implicated. The type of malignancy depends on the originating cell. The least mature lymphocytes give rise to acute lymphoblastoid leukaemia. Mature lymphocytes give rise to chronic lymphoid leukaemia or lymphoma. Tumours arising from plasma cells give rise to multiple myeloma. Each of these has unique clinical characteristics.

**38** A key characteristic of the lymphoid malignancies is that all the malignant cells will produce the same receptor or immunoglobulin. This is referred to as monoclonality. Immunological technology (electrophoresis) is used to test for monoclonal cells in samples from patients. Monoclonal animal lymphocytes are used to synthesize monoclonal antibodies, which have a range of therapeutic uses.

**39** Because immunodeficient patients are at high risk of developing some tumours, the immune system may also have a role in surveillance for malignancies. Many tumours use mechanisms for evading the immune response. Although the immune system seems unable to destroy many tumours, some tumour-effective therapies use immunological approaches.

## TRANSPLANTATION

**40** Transplantation describes the process of taking tissue or an organ from one site and placing it in another. The most commonly performed transplants are skin, kidney, heart, lung, liver, bone marrow and cornea. Autograft is the process of taking an individual's own tissue and placing it in another site in the same individual (e.g. skin grafts in patients with burns). Allograft is tissue transferred from one person to another who is genetically different. Most organ grafts are allografts.

**41** Rejection is the main problem with allografts. This is because the recipient immune system recognizes differences in the donor HLA molecules. If the recipient has antibodies against donor HLA molecules, the transplanted organ will be very rapidly destroyed: so-called hyperacute rejection. Alternatively, T cells may recognize and attack an organ when there are differences in the HLA molecules. This slower process is referred to as acute rejection.

**42** Stem cell transplant is used in the treatment of some types of malignancy and in patients with severe combined immunodeficiency (SCID). Stem cells can be obtained from donated bone marrow or blood. Transplanted stem cells may give rise to donor lymphocytes that can recognize and respond to recipient HLA. Graft-versus-host disease occurs when immunocompetent T cells in the graft tissue react to antigen on the host tissue.

**43** Tissue typing is the technology used to match recipients with donor organs. Immunosuppressive drugs are given after many forms of transplant to reduce the risk of rejection. These include tacrolimus and ciclosporin. There is a global shortage of donor organs, and genetically modified animals are being bred to overcome the problems of transplants between species (xenotransplantation).

## ■ VACCINATION

**44** Passive immunization occurs when preformed antibodies are passed to a recipient. This can occur transplacentally or through breast milk. It can also occur artificially by injection, as in the tetanus vaccine. Active immunization may occur through natural infection or by vaccination. Vaccination is the process of injecting antigen (taken from an infectious agent) into the body to raise an immune response that elicits memory T and/or B cells. The original vaccines used live organisms that had been attenuated so that they could not cause disease. These vaccines are very effective.

**45** Other vaccines contain dead organisms or subunits of organisms. These subunits are sometimes manufactured using recombinant technology. Subunit vaccines are very safe but not as effective as live vaccines. To boost their immunogenicity, subunit vaccines are generally given with an adjuvant. DNA vaccines deliver genes for pathogen proteins to elicit an immune response. Live attentuated vaccines, such as the Sabin polio vaccine, are the most effective vaccines but have the highest risk of side-effects.

## ■ IMMUNODEFICIENCY

**46** Immunodeficiency describes the state of having a reduced or defective immune component. Immuno-deficient patients are susceptible to infection by opportunistic organisms that would not normally cause disease. The exact type of organism depends on which part of the immune system is failing. Deficiencies of antibody production lead to bacterial infection while defects in T cell responses lead to infections with intracellular organisms.

**47** Antibody deficiency can be caused by defects in B cell genes and can be treated with immunoglobulin replacement.

**48** Severe combined immunodeficiency (SCID) is caused by mutations in genes that affect both T and B cells. Up to very recently, SCID has been treated with stem cell transplantation. More recently, some types of SCID have been the first diseases to be successfully treated with gene therapy.

**49** The most important cause of secondary immunodeficiency is the human immunodeficiency virus (HIV), which infects and damages T helper cells and macrophages. HIV causes a gradual decline in the immune response, especially to intracellular organisms. This leads to characteristic opportunist infections.

**50** Immunological tests (CD4 cell counts) are used to monitor HIV infection. HIV infection can be treated with antiretroviral drugs. In patients who have already become immunodeficient, antibiotics are given to prevent opportunist infections.

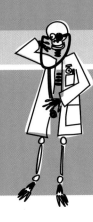

# SECTION THREE

# Fleshed out

It is very important to have a good understanding of the immune system because so many diseases are caused by immunological problems. However, many students find immunology a difficult topic and do not enjoy learning it. There are two main reasons for students struggling with immunology: some teachers get bogged down in detail of how the immune system works, without providing an overview; and some of the names of cells and molecules are very confusing.

The Big Picture is intended to make your study of the immune system easier, giving a simple overview of why we have an immune system and how the different components fit together. Make sure you have read and understood this section before moving on to the more detailed information in the Fleshed Out section.

Over the past 100 years, several thousand different immune system molecules and cells have been discovered. Fortunately, you do not need to know all of these and they can be grouped by type of activity. For the first 70 years it was not at all clear how all the different cells and molecules fitted together, so some have very strange names. For example, Toll-like receptors in humans are named after a molecule in flies called 'Toll'. In addition, molecules were given names and numbers in the order in which they were discovered, which means that the numbers often do not relate to the function of the molecules.

Some molecules have strange abbreviations, for example the CD molecules. 'CD' stands for 'cluster of differentiation' and this term was created to define specific marker molecules on the surface of cells that could be identified by a 'cluster' of techniques. As a CD marker was defined, so it was numbered. Cells expressing a given marker might have a specific function. For example, CD4 is a molecule involved in activating some T cells. All T cells that have this marker on their surface are called CD4$^+$ T cells or T helper cells.

Another strange abbreviation is IL, as in IL-1. This stands for interleukin, which were originally identified as proteins expressed by white blood cells (leukocytes) as a means of communication (inter). Now we know of many types of soluble messengers between cells (cytokines) regulating interactions in the immune system; names again have developed haphazardly and so we have abbreviations such as TNF and GM-CSF.

The questions at the start of each chapter in the Fleshed Out section will prompt you to remember the names of molecules and cells and highlight the important feature of each topic.

# 1. The barriers of the innate immune system to infection

### Questions
- What are the three characteristics of the innate immune system?
- What physical barriers does the body use to prevent infection?
- Give two examples of how flow of liquid prevents infection.

## ■ CHARACTERISTICS OF THE INNATE IMMUNE SYSTEM

The innate immune system consists of physical barriers at the surface of the body and specialized cells and molecules inside the body. The innate system has three main characteristics.

- It responds very rapidly to infection. This is because it either uses mechanisms, such as the barriers, that are present all the time, or uses cells and molecules that become active within minutes of exposure to disease-causing organisms (pathogens).
- It responds in exactly the same way each time it encounters an infection.
- It uses a handful of molecules that recognize that infection is present. These are called pattern recognition molecules.

As you learnt in The big picture, the innate immune system is very ancient. The more recently evolved adaptive immune system is described in later chapters. For the time being, make a note of the broad differences between the innate and adaptive immune systems (Table 3.1.1).

## ■ THE BODY'S BARRIERS
### Skin

The skin is the most important barrier to infection. Although there are many potential pathogens on the surface of the skin, the thick keratinized layer is impenetrable to most of these.

Injury to the skin allows pathogens to penetrate the underlying tissues. Serious burns are the most extreme example of skin injury. Patients with burns often rapidly die of overwhelming infection as vast numbers of bacteria enter the body. More usually, a minor injury only permits a small number of pathogens to enter the body and these are dealt with by other components of the innate immune system.

### The respiratory, urinary and gastrointestinal tracts

The respiratory tract, from the tip of the nose to the bronchioles, is exposed to pathogens present in the air. It is not practical to have a thickened layer of tissue similar to that in skin. Instead, the respiratory tract is lined with sticky mucus secreted by goblet cells, which traps pathogens. Underneath the mucus, the epithelial cells are covered with cilia (Fig. 3.1.1A). The beating of these cilia transports the pathogens to the pharynx or nose, where they are swallowed or sneezed out.

In cystic fibrosis, a mutation in a gene for an ion pump causes the mucus to be abnormally viscous. The mucociliary escalator cannot work normally and infections are not cleared from the lungs. Chronic lung infections are a very common cause of death in cystic fibrosis.

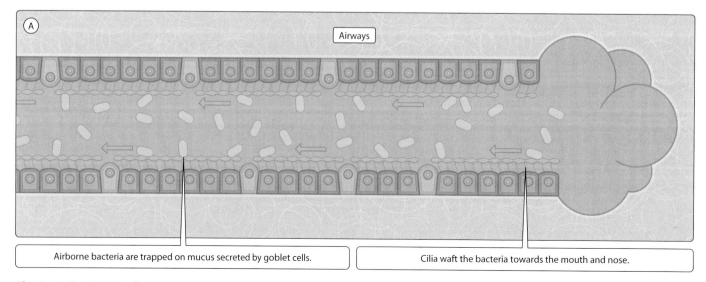

Airborne bacteria are trapped on mucus secreted by goblet cells.

Cilia waft the bacteria towards the mouth and nose.

**Fig. 3.1.1** Barriers to infection: in airways (**A**) and gastrointestinal tract (**B**, facing page).

Urine constantly flows down the urinary tract. Any pathogen would have to swim very effectively against this flow to reach the kidneys. Urinary flow can be blocked in patients who develop urinary tract stones, and pathogens often ascend as far as the kidneys in these individuals.

The majority of pathogens in food are killed by acid and proteolytic enzymes as soon as they reach the stomach. Some pathogens survive the environment of the stomach and reach the large bowel. In the large bowel, the pathogen has to compete with the many millions of faecal bacteria that normally live here. The chances of pathogens surviving this second barrier are small (Fig. 3.1.1B).

## WHY INFECTIONS OCCUR

Infection is one of the most common reasons for patients going to see doctors. Whenever they see patients with infections, it is important for doctors to consider why a patient is getting infections. Many of the clinical boxes in this book will help you to understand why patients develop infections. One very common reason for infection is that physical barriers have been damaged. Large injuries to the skin, gut or respiratory tracts almost always lead to infection.

|  | Response time | Recognition molecules | Response on repeat encounters |
|---|---|---|---|
| Innate | Seconds–minutes | Less than 30 | Unchanged |
| Adaptive | Days | More than $10^{18}$ | May be adapted |

**Table 3.1.1** The differences between the innate and adaptive immune systems.

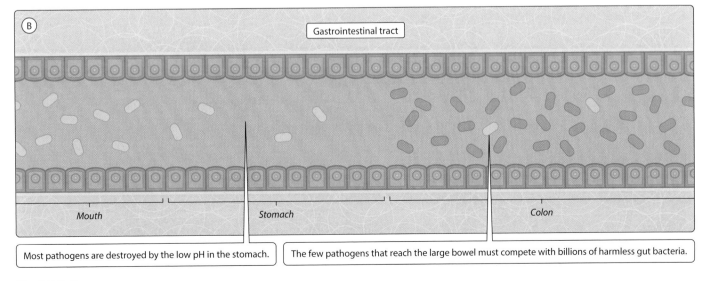

Most pathogens are destroyed by the low pH in the stomach.

The few pathogens that reach the large bowel must compete with billions of harmless gut bacteria.

**Fig. 3.1.1  B**

# 2. Pattern recognition molecules

### Questions
- How does the innate immune system recognize pathogens?
- Give examples of two different types of pattern recognition molecule.

## DETECTING INFECTION

If they are damaged, the barriers mentioned in the previous section can be breeched by pathogens. Alternatively, some pathogens have special ways of overcoming the barriers. In either case, infection then results. The innate immune system must provide a rapidly responding back-up system that operates throughout the body.

To do this, the innate immune system requires a sensory system that can detect when infection has taken place. Pattern recognition molecules recognize infection and alert the innate immune system, which then uses a range of effector systems to attack the infection.

There are differences between the metabolisms of different organisms, for example between humans and viruses. When there is a huge evolutionary gap between two species, there may be correspondingly large differences between metabolisms. For examples, many viruses produce double-stranded RNA during their life cycles. Mammalian cells never normally produce double-stranded RNA. The innate immune system uses receptors that recognize unusual pathogen-derived molecules, such as double-stranded RNA. These receptors recognize over-all patterns of molecules (for example the fact that RNA is double stranded) rather than specific features (such as the nucleotide sequence). Pattern recognition molecules also recognize that a family of pathogen is invading, such a virus, rather than a specific type of virus. The innate immune system does not, for example, distinguish between HIV and influenza.

You need to know about two types of pattern recognition molecule. The **collectins** are found in solution, while the **Toll-like receptors** (TLRs) are found on the surface of cells.

### Collectins

The collectins are a family of proteins present in solution in a range of sites throughout the body. They are called collectins because they have a *col*lagen-like region and a *lectin* region. Lectins are any protein that binds sugar molecules, usually on the surface of bacteria. Pathogens have surface sugars, for example mannose, which are absent from mammalian cell surfaces. The collagen domain interacts with the effector parts of the innate immune system.

Examples of collectins include mannose-binding lectin (MBL) and C1q, which are found in blood, and surfactant protein A, which is found in alveolar fluid.

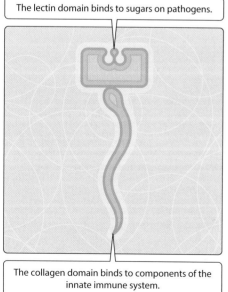
The lectin domain binds to sugars on pathogens.

The collagen domain binds to components of the innate immune system.

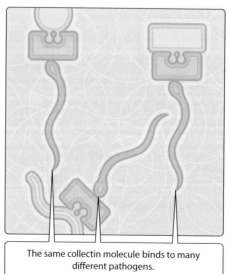
The same collectin molecule binds to many different pathogens.

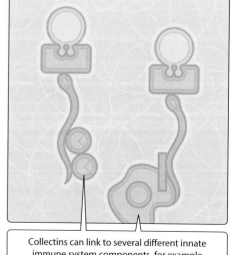
Collectins can link to several different innate immune system components, for example complement and phagocytes.

**Fig. 3.2.1** Collectins recognize many different pathogens and bind to several innate immune system molecules.

## Toll-like receptors

Toll is a molecule found in flies and forms part of the fly defence mechanism. Toll-like receptors are a family of related molecules found on the surface of mammalian cells. Each Toll-like receptor recognizes a different family of pathogen molecules. For example, TLR3 binds onto double-stranded RNA when viral infection is present. TLR4 binds a molecule called lipopolysaccharide, which is found in bacteria and fungi, but not in human cells. When the Toll-like receptors recognize pathogen molecules, they rapidly activate effector cells of the innate immune system.

 **DRUGS WHICH STIMULATE TOLL-LIKE RECEPTORS**

In several situations, it is desirable to stimulate the immune system. For example, it would be helpful to boost the immune response to cancers and some vaccines. Drugs have been developed which bind Toll-like receptors and give additional stimulus to the immune system. For example, CpG is an unmethylated DNA sequence normally only found in bacteria. CpG binds to TLR9 and by activating the immune system can be used to help to treat cancers and improve responses to vaccines.

**RECOGNITION MOLECULE LEVELS AFFECT RESISTANCE TO INFECTION**

In a population of normal people the blood level of MBL may vary up to a 1000-fold. This is because even in normal people there are differences in the exact sequence of the MBL gene. These are referred to as **polymorphisms**: genetic variation between normal members of a population. Even though people with lower levels of MBL are healthy most of the time, they are at higher risk of some infections. For example, children with low levels of MBL have a six times higher risk of developing meningococcal infection, which can cause the most severe type of meningitis.

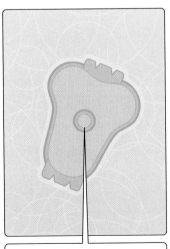

A sentinel cell resides in the tissues waiting for infection to take place.

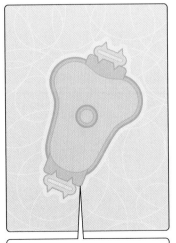

The Toll-like receptor binds a pathogen.

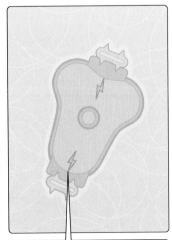

Binding activates the cell by transmitting signals to the nucleus.

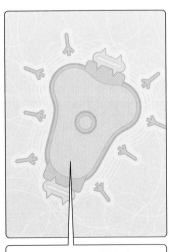

The activated cell kills the pathogen and alerts rest of the body to infection.

**Fig 3.2.2** Toll-like receptors in action.

# 3. Complement

### Questions
- Outline three ways in which complement is activated.
- Describe three effector systems of complement.
- Explain how the complement cascade amplifies signals and how it is prevented from excessive activity.

## ■ THE COMPLEMENT CASCADE

Complement comprises 20 or so blood proteins that are activated by infection and then attack pathogens. They interact with the antibodies of the adaptive immune system and were originally called complement because they complement (enhance) the effects of antibodies. We will return to this in later sections.

To understand complement, you need to remember that although there are three complement activation pathways, these all feed into one complement amplification process, and that a result of this are the actions of three different types of complement effector mechanism. The whole process is regulated by complement inhibitors.

## Complement activation pathways

The complement cascade can be activated when the collectins MBL or C1q directly bind onto pathogens (**lectin pathway**). The cascade is also activated when antibody binds C1q (**classical pathway**) (Fig. 3.3.1). MBL or C1q then forms a complex with two other components, C2 and C4. The complex C2–C4 has enzymatic activity and cleaves the next molecule, C3. C3 is typical of several of the complement proteins; it is cleaved into a large (C3b) and a small (C3a) fragment. The larger fragment, C3b, takes on enzymatic activity and activates other complement components. C3b is also able to cleave any other C3 molecules in the vicinity. C3 has a tendency to break down into C3a and C3b spontaneously (Fig. 3.3.2). This is most likely to take place on solid surfaces, for example the surface of a pathogen (**alternative pathway**).

## Complement amplification

Whichever way C3 is cleaved, it subsequently activates C5, which in turn activates C6, C7, C8 and C9. Thus a very small initial signal can end up stimulating many thousands of complement molecules. This is because several of these steps involve proteins that take on enzymatic activity and because each C3b molecule is able to cleave many more molecules of C3.

A characteristic of the complement cascade is that a very few bacterial cells can trigger a large amount of complement, because each enzyme amplifies the initial signal. The complement cascade also acts very quickly. This is important because pathogens replicate very quickly. For example, a bacterial cell

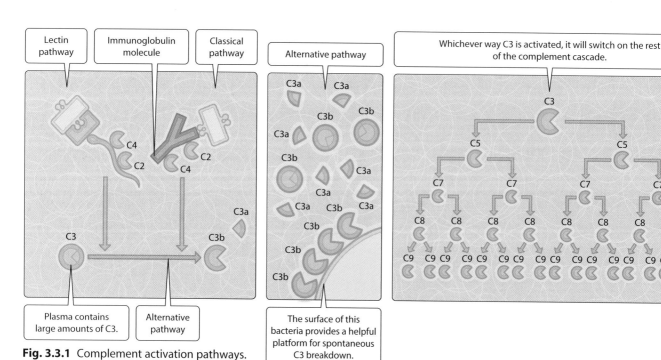

**Fig. 3.3.1** Complement activation pathways.

**Fig. 3.3.2** Activation of C3.

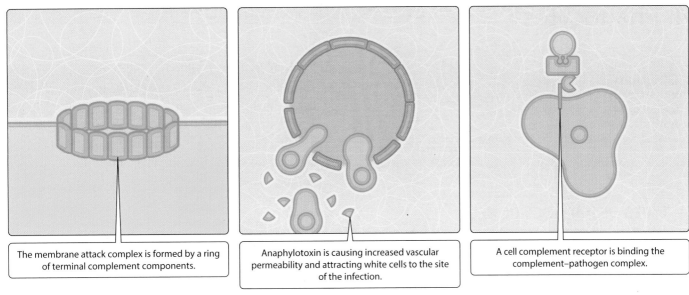

| | | |
|---|---|---|
| The membrane attack complex is formed by a ring of terminal complement components. | Anaphylotoxin is causing increased vascular permeability and attracting white cells to the site of the infection. | A cell complement receptor is binding the complement–pathogen complex. |

**Fig. 3.3.3** The consequences of complement activation.

divides every 30 minutes; within 24 hours, one bacterial cell may produce over half a million new bacteria. The result of complement activation is the direct killing of pathogens and attraction of cells to the site of infection.

## Complement effector mechanisms

Complement damages pathogens in three ways (Fig. 3.3.3):

- The final set of complement components form a polymer that binds to pathogen cell walls and punches holes in them. This is called the **membrane attack complex**.
- The low-molecular-weight fragments, for example C3a, are able to increase vascular permeability. This makes it easy for cells to approach the site of infection. These low-molecular-weight fragments are called **anaphylotoxins**.
- Other complement components stay associated with the triggering pathogens and act as bridges between cells having a receptor for complement and the pathogen.

## Complement inhibitors

Activated complement has dramatic effects and complement must be carefully controlled. The early part of the cascade is controlled by C1 inhibitor, which is normally present in the blood. Complement inhibitors are also present on the surface of normal cells, which would otherwise provide a platform for C3 cleavage.

### HEREDITARY ANGIO-OEDEMA

Hereditary angio-oedema is caused by a mutation in the C1 inhibitor gene. The early part of the complement cascade becomes activated spontaneously at times, resulting in attacks of swelling (angio-oedema). The dramatic swelling (Fig. 3.3.4) illustrates how potent the complement cascade can be when not adequately controlled. Although hereditary angio-oedema may be fatal, attacks can be treated with purified C1 inhibitor.

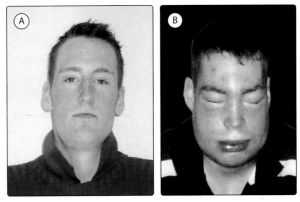

**Fig. 3.3.4** Hereditary angio-oedema. **(A)** Normal state. **(B)** During attacks the face becomes dramatically swollen.

# 4. Phagocytes

## Questions
- Describe the two main types of phagocyte.
- How are phagocytes activated?
- What is chemotaxis?
- What happens to pathogens after phagocytosis?

## ■ TYPES OF PHAGOCYTIC CELL

**Phagocytosis** is the process of a cell engulfing an object with pseudopodia so that the object is enclosed in a vacuole (a **phagosome**). There are two main types of phagocyte (Fig. 3.4.1).

- **Monocytes** are constantly produced at low levels by the bone marrow (Fig. 3.4.2). They migrate into tissues, where they mature into **macrophages**. Macrophages are sentinel cells; they survive for months or years in tissues waiting for an infection to take place. Blood filtering tissues containing high numbers of macrophages, for example the liver and spleen, are sometimes referred to as the **reticuloendothelial system.** Macrophages are also able to take on specialized forms; **osteoclasts** in bone and **glial cells** in the brain are macrophages.

- **Neutrophils** are very different. Unlike macrophages, they are not resident in normal tissues. Neutrophils only enter tissues when they are signalled to do so by macrophages. They have multilobed nuclei and cytoplasmic granules containing enzymes and defensins (Fig. 3.4.3). Once they reach the infected tissues, they only survive for a few hours or days. Because of their short lifespan, the bone marrow must produce up to 1000 billion neutrophils per day; this figure is increased during infection. Neutrophils are very mobile cells and follow trails of chemicals from the blood to the site of infection. This directional movement is called **chemotaxis**, described in detail in Chapter 23.

## ■ PHAGOCYTOSIS

Phagocytes use a variety of means to recognize pathogens, for example Toll-like receptors may recognize bacterial sugars. Pathogens that have activated the complement cascade and are coated with complement components also stimulate phagocytes. Each pathogen activates using thousands of complement molecules, making them attractive targets for phagocytes. When this has happened, the complement is said to have *opsonized* the pathogen. Both these mechanisms anchor the

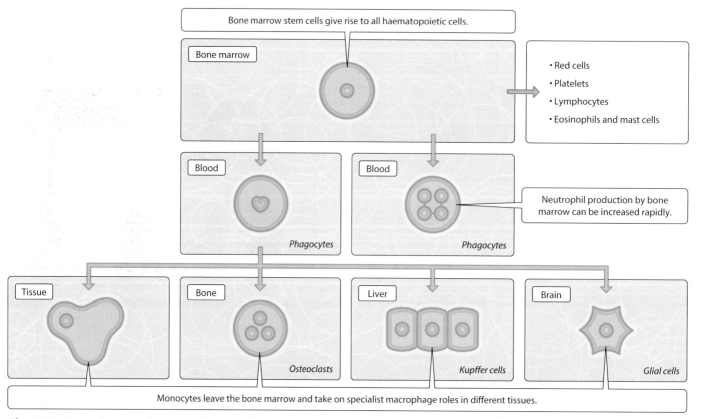

Fig. 3.4.1 Macrophages and neutrophils are both derived from the bone marrow but have very different fates.

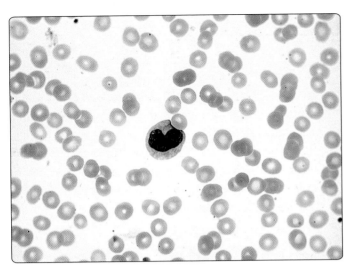

**Fig. 3.4.2** This shows a circulating monocyte in the blood. On arrival in the tissues it will mature into one of the forms of macrophage.

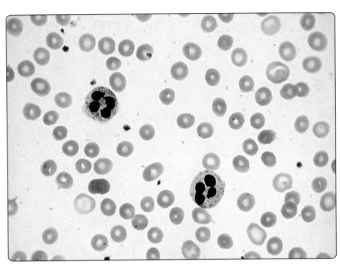

**Fig. 3.4.3** Two neutrophils in the blood: they have characteristic multilobed nuclei and their cytoplasm contains granules.

pathogen to the phagocyte and stimulate phagocytosis.

Once a pathogen is inside the phagosome, the phagocyte takes steps to kill it using several mechanisms (Fig. 3.4.4).

- The phagocyte undergoes a change in metabolism called the **respiratory burst**, which produces hypochlorous acid, hydrogen peroxide and nitric acid. Each of these chemicals can damage pathogens. Nitric acid also acts as a chemical mediator, with effects on the cardiovascular system.
- The phagocyte secretes proteolytic enzymes, which cause further damage to the pathogens.
- Defensins are secreted into the phagosome. These low-molecular-weight peptides punch holes in the pathogen cell wall.

These mechanisms kill extracellular pathogens such as bacteria and fungi. Macrophages continue to survive after phagocytosis and stimulate other components of the immune

system; this is described in the next chapter. Neutrophils are very effective at killing phagocytosed pathogens but do not survive the process. Dead neutrophils accumulate at the site of infection and produce **pus**.

### CHRONIC GRANULOMATOUS DISEASE

Some boys are born with defects in the enzymes that mediate the respiratory burst. This is caused by mutations on the X chromosome. Although neutrophils are attracted to the site of infection and phagocytose pathogens, they are unable to kill pathogens. These boys have problems with recurrent extracellular infections. This is an example of a primary immunodeficiency.

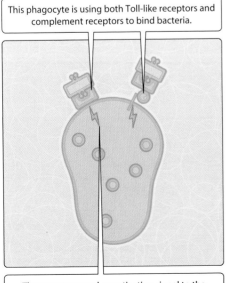

This phagocyte is using both Toll-like receptors and complement receptors to bind bacteria.

The receptors send an activating signal to the cytoplasm and nucleus.

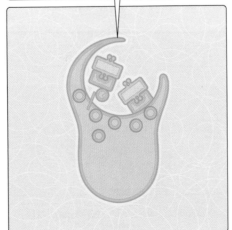

Cell cytoskeleton alters to phagocytose the bacteria and bring the granules close to the forming phagosome.

**Fig. 3.4.4** Phagocytosis.

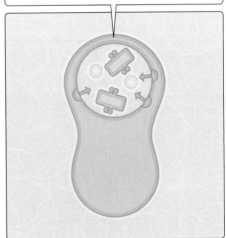

Phagosome contains discharged granule contents and newly formed hypochlorous acid, hydrogen peroxide and nitric acid.

# 5. Cytokines and the acute-phase response

## Questions
- What are cytokines?
- Give some examples of locally acting cytokines.
- How is the acute-phase response used to detect and monitor inflammation?

## ■ LOCAL EFFECTS OF MACROPHAGE CYTOKINES

Because macrophages are the first cells to recognize infection, they must alert other body systems to the presence of invaders. They do this by producing **cytokines**. Cytokines are peptide messenger molecules used for communication between cells. All the cells of the innate and adaptive immune systems can both secrete and respond to cytokines. Cytokines differ from hormones by acting both very locally and over long distances and in that they are not secreted by discrete endocrine organs. Instead, they are secreted by isolated cells situated anywhere in the body.

You have read how macrophages recruit neutrophils to the site of infection. Macrophages use three different sets of cytokines in order to do this.

1. Cytokines acting over a distance. For example, granulocyte colony-stimulating factor (G-CSF) is released by macrophages and increases the bone marrow production of neutrophils.
2. Locally acting cytokines. For example, tumour necrosis factor (TNF) acts locally to increase the stickiness of the blood vessel endothelial cells. This makes it more likely that neutrophils will then leave the blood vessels to enter surrounding tissues.
3. Chemokines (*chemo*tactic cyto*kines*) act as attractants for other cells. For example, activated macrophages release chemokines such as IL-8 that are chemotactic for neutrophils, which are guided to the site of infection (Fig. 3.5.1).

## ■ THE ACUTE-PHASE RESPONSE

The acute-phase response is a systemic, as opposed to local, reaction to infection. If an infection is not cleared, macrophage production of the cytokines IL-1, IL-6 and TNF increases and these cytokines will surge into the circulation and reach other organs (Fig. 3.5.2).

Clinical parameters that indicate infection detect the consequences of increased circulating cytokines (Fig. 3.5.3). The liver responds to these cytokines by increasing the production of a range of serum **acute-phase proteins.** C-reactive protein (CRP) is the acute-phase protein most frequently measured by clinical laboratories. CRP levels increase up to a 100-fold during infection. CRP binds to pathogens and initiates the lectin pathway of complement activation.

A side effect of the increased concentration of acute-phase proteins is that plasma viscosity increases. This is often measured in clinical laboratories as the **erythrocyte sedimentation rate** (ESR)—another marker of infection.

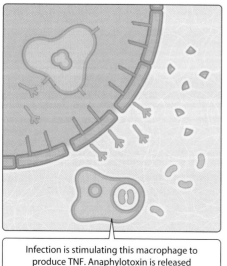

Infection is stimulating this macrophage to produce TNF. Anaphylotoxin is released by the complement cascade.

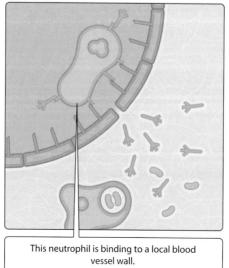

This neutrophil is binding to a local blood vessel wall.

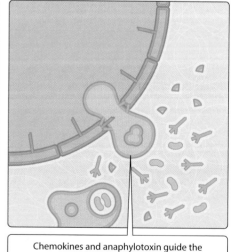

Chemokines and anaphylotoxin guide the neutrophil to the site of infection.

**Fig. 3.5.1** Cytokines collaborate with anaphylotoxin in recruiting neutrophils.

The hypothalamus has receptors for these cytokines. When these receptors are triggered, the autonomic nervous system initially responds by increasing the body temperature. Raised temperature inhibits replication of viruses and other pathogens but also acts as an important clinical clue to the presence of infection.

If the infection is not controlled at this stage, other features develop. For example the nervous system may trigger shivering and sweating: features of severe infections.

Septic shock is the most exaggerated form of acute-phase response. Very high levels of cytokines increase the production of nitric oxide, which in turn reduces cardiac output. The resultant fall in blood pressure is characteristic of very severe infections such as septicaemia.

### DIAGNOSIS OF INFECTION

A young child has been admitted to hospital with abdominal pain. At first the temperature, neutrophil count and CRP are normal. The surgeons decide to treat the child conservatively but keep her in hospital for monitoring. By the second day, she is developing an acute phase response, consistent with infection. When she is reviewed, a diagnosis of appendicitis is made and she is taken to theatre for an appendectomy.

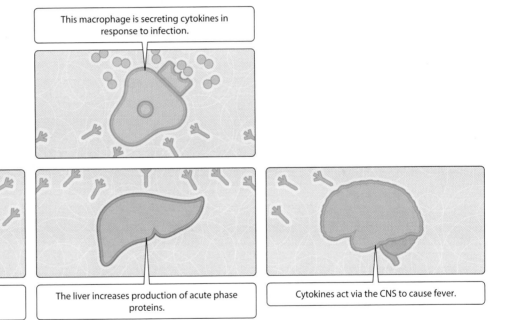

This macrophage is secreting cytokines in response to infection.

There may be an increase in pulse and fall in blood pressure.

The liver increases production of acute phase proteins.

Cytokines act via the CNS to cause fever.

**Fig. 3.5.2** The acute-phase response involves many organs.

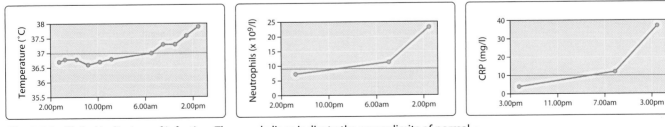

**Fig. 3.5.3** Clinical indicators of infection. The purple lines indicate the upper limits of normal.

# 6. Degranulating cells

## Questions
- Why are worms problematic and what evolved to deal with them?
- Describe the main types of degranulating cell.
- What substances are released from mast cells and eosinophils? What effects do they have?

## ■ DEALING WITH WORMS

None of the mechanisms so far described are useful for dealing with large multicellular pathogens such as worms, which are too big to be phagocytosed and may be resistant to complement. Worms are not a big problem for societies living in developed countries, but they continue to cause ill health in millions of people living in tropical, less-developed nations.

The majority of worms spend at least part of their life cycles living in the lumen of viscera such as the gut. One way of dealing with worms is to make them loosen their grip on the gut lining and then for the gut to contract, expelling the worm. These effects are mediated by degranulating cells (Fig. 3.6.1).

## ■ DEGRANULATING CELLS

Degranulating cells include **mast cells**, **basophils** and **eosinophils**. Mast cells are a little like macrophages; they are constantly present in tissues, where they have a sentinel role. Mast cells are particularly abundant in mucosal tissues. Mast cells are closely related to basophils, although the role of the latter is unclear. Eosinophils behave more like neutrophils. Eosinophils are not present in normal tissue but are recruited at times of worm infestation.

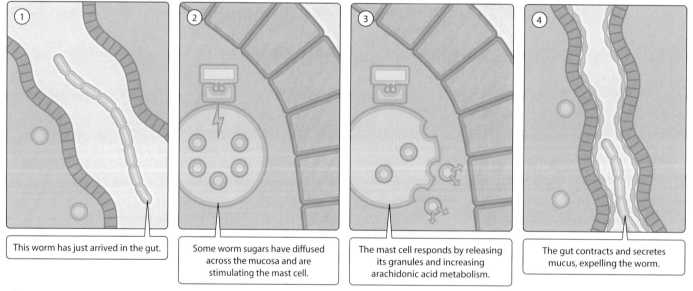

| | | | |
|---|---|---|---|
| This worm has just arrived in the gut. | Some worm sugars have diffused across the mucosa and are stimulating the mast cell. | The mast cell responds by releasing its granules and increasing arachidonic acid metabolism. | The gut contracts and secretes mucus, expelling the worm. |

**Fig. 3.6.1** Mast cells and worms

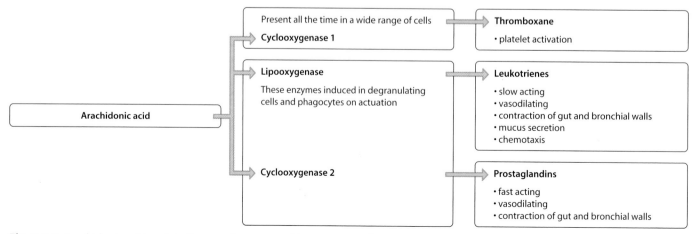

**Fig. 3.6.2** Arachidonic acid metabolism produces several important mediators.

Mast cells are probably activated when worm molecules bind to Toll-like receptors. On activation, mast cells discharge substances onto the surface of pathogens, rather than attempt to phagocytose them. Some of these substances, for example **histamine** and **proteolytic enzymes**, are preformed in resting mast cells and stored in granules. Others, for example **prostaglandins** and **leukotrienes**, are rapidly produced from arachidonic acid metabolism, after the mast cell has been activated. These substances have the following effects:

- histamine causes contraction of smooth muscle in the gut and airways and relaxation of smooth muscle around blood vessels
- proteolytic enzymes, for example mast cell tryptase, can cleave C3 and activate the complement pathway
- arachidonic acid metabolites (thromboxane, leukotrienes, prostaglandins) have multiple actions (Fig. 3.6.2)

- cytokines such as IL-3 and IL-8 activate eosinophils and adaptive immune system cells.

The net effect of these mediators is that mucus secretion increases and smooth muscle contracts; this may be enough to expel the worm. In addition, blood vessels become dilated and other white cells are attracted by chemotaxis to the site of worm infestation. This recruitment is similar to macrophages attracting neutrophils to the site of a bacterial infection.

One of the cell types recruited to the site of worm infestation is eosinophils (Fig. 3.6.3). Eosinophil production in the bone marrow is increased by IL-3 and IL-5. Leukotrienes are chemotractant for eosinophils and draw them to the site of worm infestation.

Eosinophils release similar substances to mast cells (except histamine). In addition they release three very noxious substances:

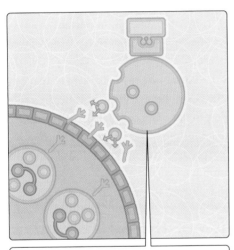

This activated mast cell is secreting IL-3. Eosinophil numbers have increased.

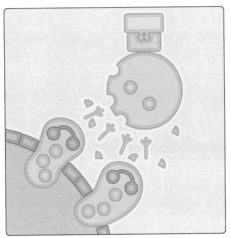

Prostaglandin and C3a increase blood vessel permeability and are chemotactic for eosinophils.

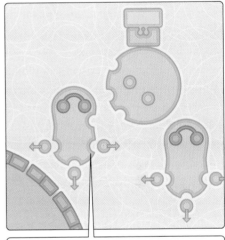

Activated eosinophils release extra mediators.

**Fig. 3.6.3** Activated mast cells recruit eosinophils to the site of worm infestation.

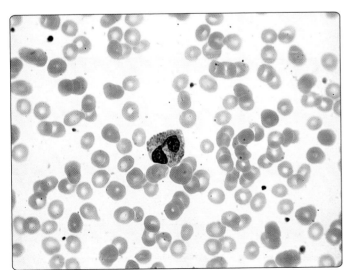

**Fig. 3.6.4** An esinophil in the blood. It has red granules, compared with the blue granules seen in neutrophils (Fig. 3.4.3).

- a peroxidase that generates hypochlorous acid
- a basic protein that attacks the outer layers of the parasite
- a cationic protein that also damages the worm's outer layers and paralyses its nervous system.

Mast cells, but not eosinophils, can also be activated when an antibody called IgE is bound to their surface. Although IgE probably evolved to facilitate worm expulsion, it also causes allergies. This important mechanism will be explained in Chapter 28.

 **EOSINOPHILIA**

People who live in areas where worm infestation is common have high numbers of eosinophils in their blood (Fig. 3.6.4). In the developed world, eosinophilia is more likely to be a sign of severe allergies.

# 7. Interferons and other danger signals

**Questions**
- How and when are interferons secreted?
- What are the actions of interferons?
- Describe some innate immune system danger signals.

## INTRACELLULAR PATHOGENS

A variety of organisms have adapted themselves for life inside cells. True intracellular organisms live inside the cytoplasm or nucleus; these include all viruses and some protozoans. All viruses spend part of their life cycles inside host cells. Some bacteria (especially *Mycobacterium* spp.) are phagocytosed but cannot be destroyed in the process. Mycobacteria have waxy coats that are resistant to the proteolytic enzymes present in phagosomes. All these organisms are resistant to all the killing mechanisms so far described.

The innate immune system can inhibit replication of some intracellular pathogens by secreting interferons. Interferons are so called because when first discovered they were shown to be able to interfere with viral replication. Interferons $\alpha$ and $\beta$ have strong antiviral effects; interferon $\gamma$ is only weakly antiviral. Interferon $\gamma$ has a more important role in cross-talk between T cells of the adaptive immune system and macrophages.

## INTERFERON $\alpha$ AND $\beta$

Cells use innate mechanisms to recognize that intracellular viral infection is taking place. For example, TLR3 can recognize double-stranded RNA, the presence of which suggests that viral infection is taking place. In response, the stimulated cell secretes interferons $\alpha$ and $\beta$ (Fig. 3.7.1).

Interferons $\alpha$ and $\beta$ are secreted by a wide range of cells and can be produced very rapidly at the site where the virus enters the body.

Interferons do not destroy viruses, but they do prevent viruses from replicating. They do this by activating an enzyme called oligo-adenylate synthase, which degrades viral RNA. Interferons also switch off protein synthesis, which prevents viral replication. These effects of interferon can be very local. However, interferons $\alpha$ and $\beta$ stimulate other innate and adaptive immune system cells to make certain the response to viral infection is effective. This is one example of the innate immune system providing a 'danger signal' of infection. These interferons also activate dendritic cells, which have an important role in stimulating the adaptive system. Finally, interferons can activate the acute phase response.

Each component of the innate systems sends signals that can spread further across the body. These signals activate the acute phase response and also provide 'danger signals' to alert further components of the innate immune system and of the adaptive immune system to the presence of infection (Fig. 3.7.2). In general, the adaptive immune system will not respond unless it has received a danger signal from the innate system.

## A QUICK REVIEW OF THE INNATE IMMUNE SYSTEM

We have now reached the end of the section on the innate immune system and will next move on to the adaptive immune

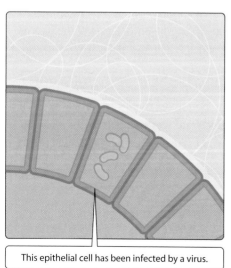
This epithelial cell has been infected by a virus.

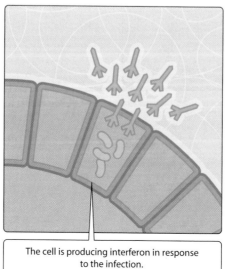
The cell is producing interferon in response to the infection.

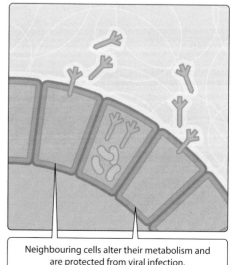
Neighbouring cells alter their metabolism and are protected from viral infection.

**Fig. 3.7.1** Interferon is secreted in response to viral infection.

system. The innate immune system is able to kill many pathogens effectively and is so important that you would rapidly die without it. For example, if you had severe burns and your skin was extensively damaged, you would soon be overwhelmed by infection. Or if your bone marrow was damaged by radiation or drugs and was unable to produce the 1000 billion neutrophils it normally produces each day, you would die of infection within a few hours.

However, there are limitations to what the innate immune system can do. For example, interferons can stop viral replication, but they do not actually kill viruses that have invaded the body. The same is true for bacteria that have

evolved to live inside cells. Intracellular pathogens cannot be killed by interferons and so specialized mechanisms are needed to kill them; these are the cytotoxic T cells of the adaptive immune system.

The second problem with the innate immune system is that, even though it can respond quickly, it does require the presence of quite a few pathogens (and hence some pathogen replication) before it becomes activated. The adaptive immune system produces long-lasting antibodies, which are present on mucosal surfaces and in the blood before re-exposure to a pathogen. Antibodies provide immunological memory and instantaneous protection against some infections.

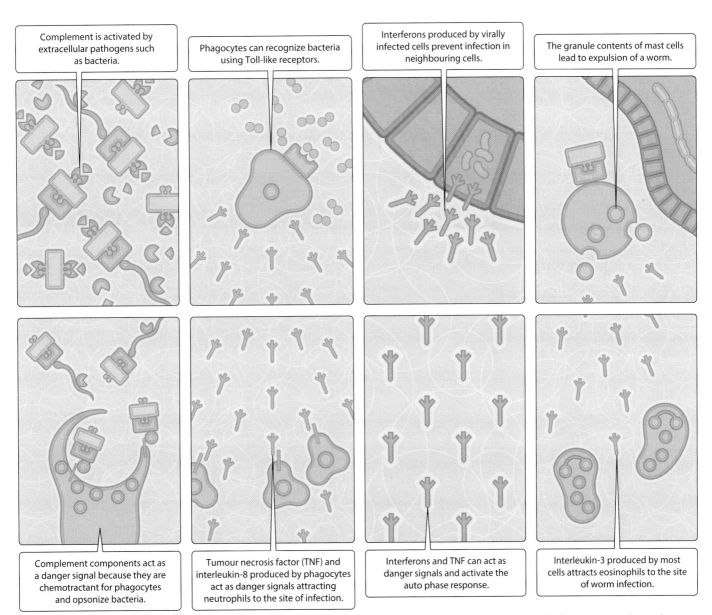

**Fig. 3.7.2** The top row shows innate immune system components detecting and dealing with infection. The bottom row shows the danger signals each component produces.

# 8. Peptide antigen processing and display

### Questions
- What is an antigen?
- Describe how peptide antigens are produced by two different pathways.
- What are the characteristics of the immunoglobulin superfamily?
- Describe the function of HLA class I and class II.

## ■ INTRACELLULAR AND PHAGOCYTOSED ANTIGEN

Antigens are substances that are recognized by the specific receptors of the adaptive immune system. These receptors are the T cell receptor and immunoglobulin; you will read a lot more about these in the next 12 chapters. Most antigens are specific for the pathogen from which they were derived. For example, although both HIV and influenza are viruses, they produce very different antigens.

T cells recognize peptide antigens derived from the intracellular pathogens and pathogens inside phagosomes, described in the previous chapters. T cells have no way of looking directly into infected cells. Peptide antigen must be processed from the pathogen deep inside the cell, bought to the cell surface and then bound to the cell surface. Apart from being bound to the cell surface, special molecules are required to alert T cells to the fact that an antigen from inside the cell is being presented. The two processes required to do this are **antigen processing**, whereby small **peptide antigens** are produced and moved to the cell surface, and **antigen display**, whereby antigen is held there (Fig. 3.8.1). These processes differ for true intracellular pathogens and for pathogens held in phagosomes.

## Processing and display of antigen from intracellular pathogens

Proteosomes are collections of proteolytic enzymes found in the cytoplasm. They digest the proteins that make up intracellular pathogen, producing small peptides 8–15 amino acid residues long. Proteosomes become more active when the cell has been activated by interferons. **T**ransport associated with **a**ntigen **p**rocessing (TAP) pumps these peptides across the cytoplasm into the endoplasmic reticulum.

Peptides produced by antigen processing are held on the cell surface in a groove along the surface of **HLA** molecules (the human MHC system is known as HLA (human leukocyte antigen)). HLA is a member of the **immunoglobulin super-family** of proteins (Fig. 3.8.2). Peptides from intracellular pathogens are bound to HLA class I. HLA class I has two peptides: the α chain has three domains and the smaller β chain

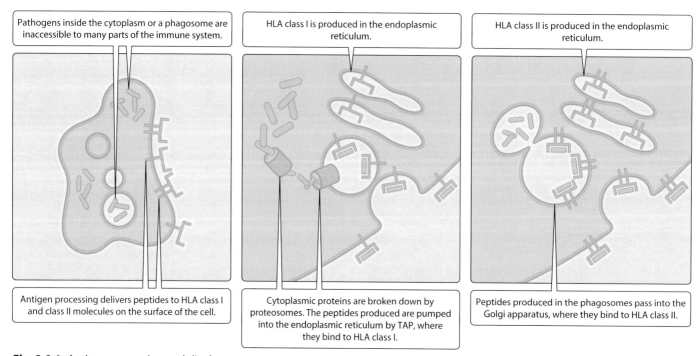

Pathogens inside the cytoplasm or a phagosome are inaccessible to many parts of the immune system.

HLA class I is produced in the endoplasmic reticulum.

HLA class II is produced in the endoplasmic reticulum.

Antigen processing delivers peptides to HLA class I and class II molecules on the surface of the cell.

Cytoplasmic proteins are broken down by proteosomes. The peptides produced are pumped into the endoplasmic reticulum by TAP, where they bind to HLA class I.

Peptides produced in the phagosomes pass into the Golgi apparatus, where they bind to HLA class II.

**Fig. 3.8.1** Antigen processing and display.

has a single domain; the latter molecule is known as **$\beta_2$-microglobulin**. Helical amino acid sequences in the $\alpha_1$ and $\alpha_2$ domains form the side of the antigen peptide-binding groove. Some peptides produced from cytoplasmic proteins will fit into the groove. The HLA–peptide is then displayed on the surface of the cell.

## Processing and display of antigen from pathogens held in phagosomes

Proteolytic enzymes in the phagosome digest extracellular pathogens that have been phagocytosed. The peptides produced pass from the phagosome to the interconnecting Golgi apparatus, where they are bound to HLA class II molecules. The class II molecules are made up of two chains, $\alpha$ and $\beta$, each made up of two immunoglobulin-like domains. The $\alpha_1$ and $\beta_1$ chain domains contain helices, which form the two sides of the antigen-binding groove.

## Identifying pathogen proteins

A very important concept is that peptide antigens from intracellular pathogens are directed to HLA class I molecules, while peptide antigens from material in phagosomes is associated with HLA class II molecules. The type of HLA a peptide antigen is bound to on the cell surface indicates its origin. It is also important to understand that these sampling processes are random. It is quite possible that normal self-proteins could be broken down by either pathway and that

normal self-peptides could end up being displayed on the HLA molecules. The sampling mechanisms cannot distinguish between self-proteins and pathogen proteins and peptides. This distinction is left to T cells, which are selected on the basis that they will not respond to self-peptides.

### THE IMMUNOGLOBULIN SUPERFAMILY

The members of the immunoglobulin superfamily are all proteins made of globular domains, linked by shorter flexible peptide sequences and stabilized by disulphide bonds. All these molecules are expressed at the surface of cells but have tails which are anchored in the cytoplasm. Most of these molecules are involved in communication between different cells.

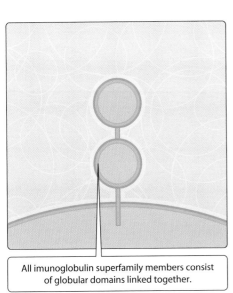
All imunoglobulin superfamily members consist of globular domains linked together.

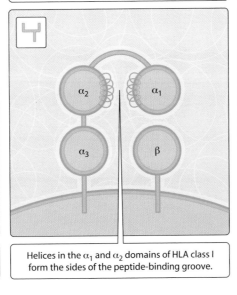
HLA class I

Helices in the $\alpha_1$ and $\alpha_2$ domains of HLA class I form the sides of the peptide-binding groove.

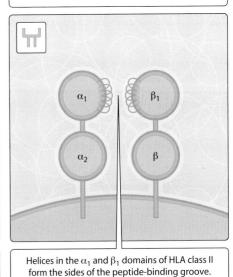
HLA class II

Helices in the $\alpha_1$ and $\beta_1$ domains of HLA class II form the sides of the peptide-binding groove.

**Fig. 3.8.2** Structure of HLA.

# 9. The T cell receptor and the generation of diversity

## Questions
- What is the structure of the T cell receptor?
- Why is gene recombination, rather than gene duplication, required to generate T cell receptor genes?
- What is meant by polyclonality?

## ■ STRUCTURE OF THE T CELL RECEPTOR

T cells use a **T cell receptor** to recognize antigen specifically. The T cell receptor must recognize simultaneously both the peptide antigen and the HLA molecule it is lying in. This is why the T cell receptor only recognizes intracellular or phagocytosed antigen. This section explains how a specific T cell receptor is generated for the vast number of peptide antigens created by processing.

The T cell receptor is a dimer of two immunoglobulin superfamily molecule chains. Over 95% of T cells use one α and one β chain. T cells using γ and δ chains are much rarer and are mentioned in Chapter 22.

The α and β chains each consist of two domains. The constant domain, closest to the cell surface, is the same in all T cells. The variable domain is further away and comes into contact with antigen and HLA (Fig. 3.9.1). Part of the variable domain is referred to as the hypervariable region. The amino acid sequences in this region vary considerably from T cell to T cell. The hypervariable region binds to antigen, and the very high variability enables any given T cell receptor to be specific for a peptide antigen.

## ■ GENERATION OF DIVERSITY

Each peptide antigen consists of at least eight amino acid residues. There are 20 amino acids available, so there are at least $2.6 \times 10^{10}$ ($20^8$) possible peptide antigens. One way to deal with this huge number of possible peptide antigens would be to have entirely separate genes for each T cell receptor. These genes would have the same basic framework but differ slightly in the antigen-binding region. This is called gene duplication and is used by the HLA system to produce a limited amount of diversity in each individual. Each cell contains genes for up to 12 different HLA molecules. The human genome only has room for about 30 000 genes, so even if all of these were used for T cell receptors, gene duplication would not provide enough genes for all the T cell receptors required (Fig. 3.9.2).

To overcome the lack of space on the genome, the T cell receptor genes use *genetic recombination* to produce the diversity of receptors required. T cell receptor and immunoglobulin genes are the only human genes to undergo recombination.

The gene for each receptor consists of gene segments for the constant domain and for the variable domain. The constant

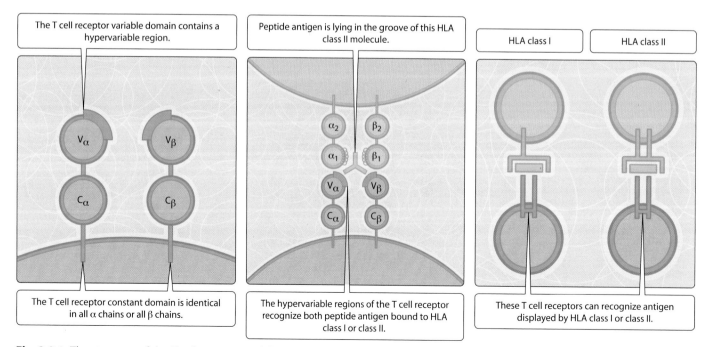

The T cell receptor variable domain contains a hypervariable region.

Peptide antigen is lying in the groove of this HLA class II molecule.

HLA class I    HLA class II

$V_\alpha$    $V_\beta$

$C_\alpha$    $C_\beta$

$\alpha_2$    $\beta_2$
$\alpha_1$    $\beta_1$
$V_\alpha$    $V_\beta$
$C_\alpha$    $C_\beta$

The T cell receptor constant domain is identical in all α chains or all β chains.

The hypervariable regions of the T cell receptor recognize both peptide antigen bound to HLA class I or class II.

These T cell receptors can recognize antigen displayed by HLA class I or class II.

**Fig. 3.9.1** The structure of the T cell receptor and the relationship to HLA.

domain gene segments are like segments of normal genes: there is one copy of the gene segment for each α or β chain constant region. The gene segments for the variable region are very different. There are multiple copies of two (for the α chain) or three (for the β chain) hypervariable region gene segments. One copy from each segment is randomly cut and pasted to create up to $10^{12}$ different T cell receptor genes. The details of T cell receptor gene recombination are covered in the next chapter.

## CLONALITY

In a healthy individual, T cells in the blood express several million different types of receptor. Hidden in the overall T cell population, there may be small families of cells with identical receptors. These families are called **clones** and are derived from the same predecessor cell. This situation of many different clones expressing different receptors is referred to as **polyclonality**. If you were to look at a random selection of blood T cells, the chances are they would have different receptors.

In a viral infection, Th1 cells stimulate the dramatic proliferation of cytotoxic T cells specific for the viral antigens. The blood will have many copies of T cells carrying the same T cell receptors (clones) and this is often referred to as **oligoclonality**. A blood sample might show just a few dominant T cell receptors being used.

**Monoclonality** occurs when there is only a single T cell receptor (or immunoglobulin) and is often seen in lymphoid malignancies. A blood sample would show that all the T cells are using exactly the same receptor.

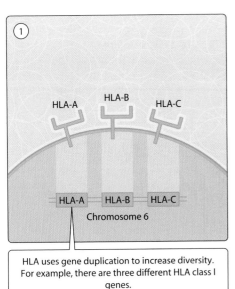

HLA uses gene duplication to increase diversity. For example, there are three different HLA class I genes.

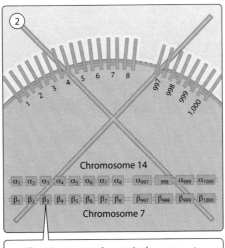

There is not enough room in the genome to include different genes for the α and β chains of every T cell receptor required.

T cell receptors use gene recombination to increase diversity. There are between 2 and 80 gene segments for the hypervariable region, which can be cut and pasted together.

**Fig. 3.9.2** Gene duplication allows for several HLA genes. Gene recombination is required to create the billions of T cell receptor genes.

# 10. T cell receptor gene recombination

## Questions
- What are the steps of genetic recombination?
- What other two mechanisms are used to introduce diversity to T cell receptor genes?
- What are the dangers of recombination?

## ■ THE T CELL RECEPTOR GENES

The adaptive immune system uses genetic recombination (also called rearrangement) to generate additional genetic sequences because there is not enough room in the genome for individual genes for each receptor required. Recombination is the rearrangement of a limited number of existing gene segments to create a much greater number of new sequences.

Before recombination, the gene segments are all present in the **germline configuration**. The α and β chains of the T cell receptor each contain only one constant domain gene segment. Recombination is only used to produce variation in the variable domain. The recombination process is simpler for the α chain gene variable region. The α chain variable domain is encoded by a V (variable) gene segment and a J gene segment (joining gene; it connects the variable and constant domain). One of 50 V gene segments and one of 70 J gene segments are used to encode the α variable domain. Exactly which of these V and J gene segments

are used happens at random: the T cell does not choose which genes to use. The gene segments that are not used are cut out of the sequence and the newly configured gene is transcribed and translated in the normal way (Fig. 3.10.1).

The β chain is slightly more complex. In addition to 57 V gene segments and 13 J gene segments, there are two D (diversity) gene segments, one of which is also used. Once again, one V, one D and one J gene segments are used at random to produce a new sequence.

## ■ ENZYMES CREATING DIVERSITY

V(D)J recombinase is a family of enzymes responsible for recombining both T cell receptor and immunoglobulin genes. The process is initiated by recombinase enzymes recognizing sequences at random 3′ ends of the V or D gene segment and the 5′ ends of the D or J segments. The DNA is cut and the unused gene segments are removed as **excision circles**. The DNA cutting is not precise and may remove extra nucleotides from one or other DNA strand (Fig. 3.10.2).

In addition, an enzyme called **terminal deoxynucleotide transferase** (TdT) adds random base pairs to the cut ends. Once recombinase enzymes have joined the two ends, the base pair substitutions induced by TdT and uneven cutting have the effect of changing the base pair sequence in the recombined gene (Fig. 3.10.3).

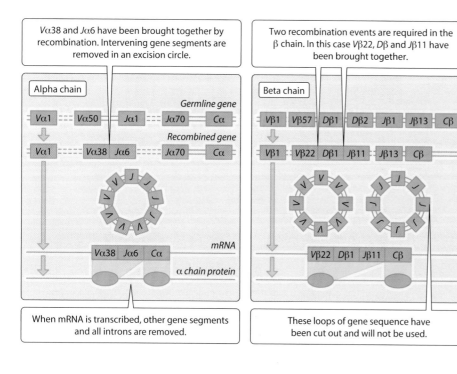

Vα38 and Jα6 have been brought together by recombination. Intervening gene segments are removed in an excision circle.

Two recombination events are required in the β chain. In this case Vβ22, Dβ and Jβ11 have been brought together.

When mRNA is transcribed, other gene segments and all introns are removed.

These loops of gene sequence have been cut out and will not be used.

**Fig. 3.10.1** Gene segments are used to generate the α and β chains of the T cell receptor.

T cell receptor diversity is consequently generated by two different phases:

1. recombination of gene segments, leading to $5.2 \times 10^6$ possible variants
2. changes in base pair sequences at the DNA joining site, adding $3 \times 10^6$ variants.

Together, these processes allow for $1.56 \times 10^{13}$ different T cell receptors, which are easily enough to deal with the $2.6 \times 10^{10}$ possible peptide antigens generated by processing.

Genetic recombination is a good way of creating new genes for millions of different molecules, but it is only used by the T and B cells of the immune system. This is because recombination is potentially a very dangerous process. Recombination could lead to malignancy if oncogenes were inadvertently affected. In addition, recombination could generate receptors that recognize normal host tissues.

## RECOMBINASE DEFECTS

Some children are born with defects in the recombinase enzymes. These children cannot produce T or B cells and experience severe infections from birth. This and primary immunodeficiency are discussed in Chapter 48.

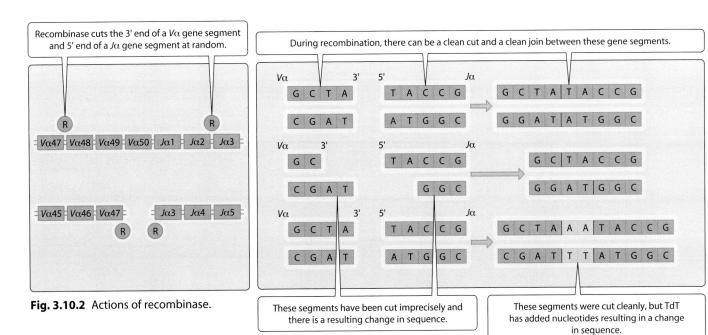

**Fig. 3.10.2** Actions of recombinase.

**Fig. 3.10.3** Further diversity is created by changing the nucleotide sequence at the joined ends.

# 11. T cell activation

## Questions
- Contrast the two different types of T cell.
- What is the immunological synapse?
- Describe how surface events involving CD3, CD4 and CD8 are linked to gene transcription.

## WHEN DO T CELLS BECOME ACTIVATED?

T cells recognize infection by binding intracellular or phagocytosed peptide antigen lying in the groove of HLA. The T cell receptor specifically binds antigen and the HLA molecule.

The result of T cell receptor binding to antigen can be gene transcription and T cell proliferation. This chapter discusses intracellular signalling; how messages from the T cell receptor increase the transcription of genes in the nucleus. Before you read about signalling, you need to know more about two different types of T cell.

### T cell subsets

As described in previous sections, peptides from intracellular proteins are displayed on HLA class I and peptides from phagocytosed proteins are displayed on class II. Each of these types of peptide is recognized by a different subset of T cell.

- **Cytotoxic T cells** recognize intracellular infection, in which case the antigenic peptide is bound to HLA class I. Cytotoxic T cells express a molecule called CD8, which specifically recognizes HLA class I. The role of cytotoxic T cells is to kill infected cells.
- **Helper T cells** recognize antigenic peptides generated in the phagosome and bound to HLA class II. Helper T cells use a molecule called CD4 to recognize HLA class II. Helper T cells coordinate the immune response.

## INTRACELLULAR SIGNALLING

CD3, CD8 and CD4 are the surface molecules that initiate intracellular signalling following T cell receptor binding to antigen. The T cell receptor, CD3 and CD8 or CD4 are normally spread evenly across the T cell surface and do not interact. These molecules are drawn together to form an **immunological synapse** when they encounter a cell with antigen in the groove of its HLA molecules (an **antigen-presenting cell**). The cytoplasmic tails of CD3, CD4 and CD8 contain regions that can activate intracellular kinase enzymes but only when these molecules are collected together in sufficient density (Fig. 3.11.1).

The immunological synapse formed in response to antigen presentation initiates a series of intracellular changes leading to

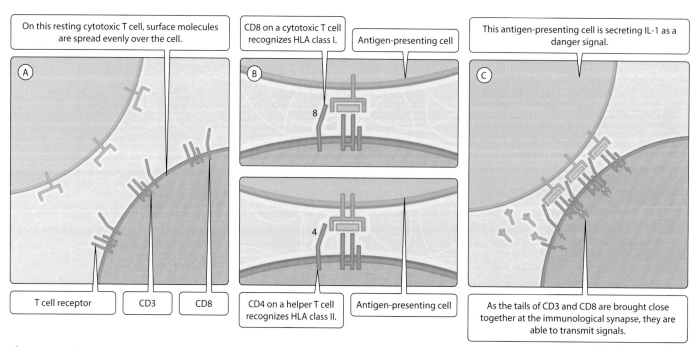

**Fig. 3.11.1** The signalling events in CD8+ and CD4+ T cells are very similar.

gene transcription (Fig. 3.11.2). Several kinases are involved in T cell signalling. Each kinase phosphorylates and activates further kinases. The kinases involved in intracellular signalling in T cells form a cascade; each activated kinase is able to activate many more; as a result, the initial small signal at the cell surface is amplified many times. Increased kinase activity causes transcription factors to move from the cytoplasm to the nucleus. In the nucleus, transcription factors bind to the enhancers and promoters of genes and increase their transcription. NFAT and NF-κB are examples of transcription factors with a special role in T cells.

Another consequence of kinase activation is that calcium ions flow into the T cell. The increased concentration of calcium activates a family of proteins called **immunophilins**, which also activate transcription factors.

One outcome of gene transcription is secretion of the lymphocyte growth factor IL-2. IL-2 secretion commits the T cell and its neighbours to proliferation. However, other outcomes, including T cell death, can also occur after signalling through the T cell receptor. The exact outcome of T cell receptor signalling depends on when and how it takes place.

## THERAPEUTIC SUPPRESSION OF THE IMMUNE SYSTEM

It is often desirable to switch off the immune system, for example during organ transplantation. Ciclosporin and tacrolimus are immunosuppressive drugs that bind to immunophylin, preventing it from activating T cell transcription factors.

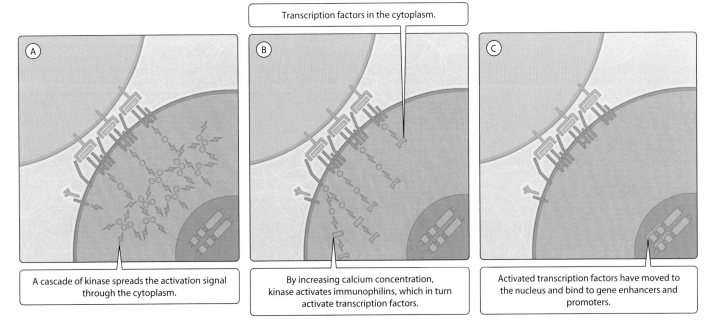

Transcription factors in the cytoplasm.

A — A cascade of kinase spreads the activation signal through the cytoplasm.

B — By increasing calcium concentration, kinase activates immunophilins, which in turn activate transcription factors.

C — Activated transcription factors have moved to the nucleus and bind to gene enhancers and promoters.

**Fig. 3.11.2** Events leading to gene transcription in the T cell.

# 12. T cell tolerance and the thymus

## Questions
- What is meant by self-restriction and self-tolerance?
- Contrast the different aims and mechanisms of positive and negative selection.
- What is T cell tolerance?
- How is tolerance achieved outside the thymus?
- What is anergy?

## ■ THE THYMUS

T cells develop in the thymus in late fetal life and throughout childhood. The thymus stops producing new T cells in adolescence, after which T cell numbers are maintained by proliferation outside the thymus, in the periphery.

The thymus uses two criteria to select T cells that are allowed to pass on to the periphery.

1. T cells must recognize either self-HLA class I (using CD8) or self-HLA class II (using CD4). These cells are selected for being **self-restricted** and are selected through **positive selection**.

2. Normal self-peptides constantly enter the antigen-presenting pathways. These self-peptides must not be recognized by T cells. T cells that have been selected because they do not to recognize self-peptides are described as being **self-tolerant** and are selected through **negative selection**.

These two steps take place one after the other in the thymic cortex and medulla, respectively.

## Positive selection

Pre-T cells migrate from the liver to the thymus. Inside the thymus, these cells are called thymocytes and express T cell receptors and both CD8 and CD4. In the thymic cortex, when the T cell receptor recognizes self-HLA on thymic epithelium, it transmits a signal that allows the cell to survive. T cells that do not recognize self-HLA die. This process is called positive selection. At the same time, T cells that recognize HLA class I lose CD4 and those that recognize HLA class II lose CD8. The resulting populations of T cells are thus selected for HLA class I (CD8+ cells) or HLA class II (CD4+ cells) (Fig. 3.12.1).

## Negative selection

The thymocytes move to the thymic medulla and encounter dendritic cells. These cells actively sample and display a wide range of normal self-peptides from the environment and from the cytoplasm.

In the thymic medulla, when the T cell receptor recognizes self-peptides and HLA it transmits a signal that forces the cell to die. Thus, T cells that are capable of recognizing self-peptides plus HLA are deleted through negative selection (Fig. 3.12.2A).

Over 90% of thymocytes die during positive and negative selection. This includes cells that *do not* receive a T cell receptor

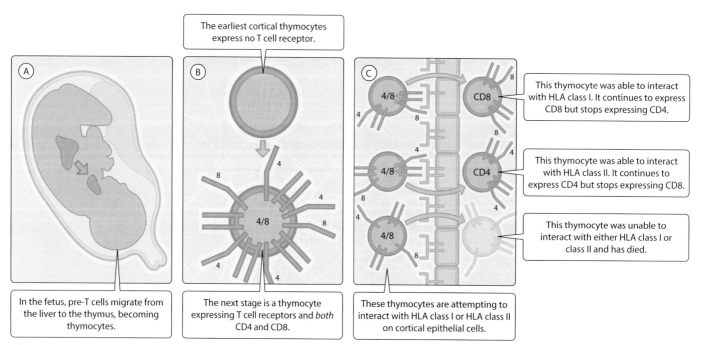

The earliest cortical thymocytes express no T cell receptor.

This thymocyte was able to interact with HLA class I. It continues to express CD8 but stops expressing CD4.

This thymocyte was able to interact with HLA class II. It continues to express CD4 but stops expressing CD8.

This thymocyte was unable to interact with either HLA class I or class II and has died.

In the fetus, pre-T cells migrate from the liver to the thymus, becoming thymocytes.

The next stage is a thymocyte expressing T cell receptors and *both* CD4 and CD8.

These thymocytes are attempting to interact with HLA class I or HLA class II on cortical epithelial cells.

**Fig. 3.12.1** Positive selection.

signal in the thymic cortex and cells that *do* receive a signal in the thymic medulla. The cells that die commit suicide through a process called **apoptosis**, which you will read more about in Chapter 14. The result of positive and negative selection is CD8+ T cells (which can recognize intracellular infection) and CD4+ T cells (which can recognize antigens from phagosomes) (Fig. 3.12.2B).

## T CELL TOLERANCE

Tolerance is the state in which clones of T cells do not recognize self-antigen. In the thymus, this is bought about by negative selection. Induction of tolerance by the thymus is not 100% effective and some self-reactive T cells escape into the periphery, where they could cause damage. **Peripheral tolerance** is the final check to this. T cells that react to antigen and HLA in the absence of a danger signal (such as the cytokine IL-1) provided by the innate immune system do not become activated. Instead, they become **anergic**, which means they become permanently dormant and cannot respond to antigen again (Fig. 3.12.3). The results of stimulation through the T cell receptor depend on exactly how and where the cell is being stimulated.

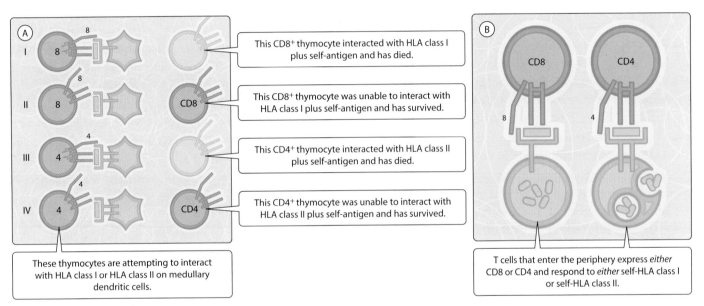

This CD8+ thymocyte interacted with HLA class I plus self-antigen and has died.

This CD8+ thymocyte was unable to interact with HLA class I plus self-antigen and has survived.

This CD4+ thymocyte interacted with HLA class II plus self-antigen and has died.

This CD4+ thymocyte was unable to interact with HLA class II plus self-antigen and has survived.

These thymocytes are attempting to interact with HLA class I or HLA class II on medullary dendritic cells.

T cells that enter the periphery express *either* CD8 or CD4 and respond to *either* self-HLA class I or self-HLA class II.

**Fig. 3.12.2** Negative selection.

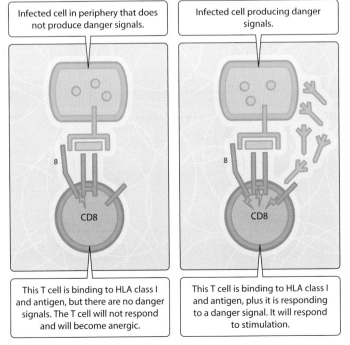

Infected cell in periphery that does not produce danger signals.

Infected cell producing danger signals.

This T cell is binding to HLA class I and antigen, but there are no danger signals. The T cell will not respond and will become anergic.

This T cell is binding to HLA class I and antigen, plus it is responding to a danger signal. It will respond to stimulation.

**Fig. 3.12.3** Peripheral tolerance.

### THE DI GEORGE SYNDROME

In the Di George syndrome, the thymus is absent. These children can have very low numbers of T cells and suffer from severe infections.

# 13. HLA restriction and polymorphism

## Questions
- Why have humans evolved polymorphic HLA genes?
- Describe how there is limited HLA variation in an individual, but wide variation in a population?
- What are antigen-presenting cells?

## ■ THE MHC

The **major histocompatibility complex** (MHC) is a cluster of genes named because they determine whether transplanted tissue is compatible between donor and host. This cluster occurs in all vertebrates. The system in humans is called the HLA but HLA and MHC are sometimes used interchangeably.

There are three different genes for the α chains of HLA class I molecules (HLA-A, HLA-B and HLA-C) and three different sets of genes for the α and β chains of class II (HLA-DP, HLA-DQ and HLA-DR). HLA genes are co-dominant; each inherited gene is expressed. This means that a total of 12 maternal and paternal genes are expressed. The HLA genes from each parent are inherited in a block called a **haplotype** (Fig. 3.13.1).

HLA class I is expressed on all nucleated cells and displays peptide derived from intracellular infections to cytotoxic (CD8⁺) T cells. HLA class II is normally only expressed on a few cells, for example macrophages, dendritic cells and B cells. These cells very effectively process extracellular pathogens and display peptides on class II to helper (CD4⁺) T cells. They are sometimes referred to as antigen-presenting cells.

## ■ HLA POLYMORPHISM

The groove of any HLA class I or class II molecule is narrow and crooked and only some peptides can fit into it, depending on their precise amino acid sequence. As a result, any given HLA molecule is only able to bind a few different peptides. Although each individual has genes for 12 different HLA molecules, they are only able to bind a minority of all the potential peptides that could be derived from pathogens.

To overcome the constraint the number of HLA genes would place on peptide binding, the genes have become polymorphic. **Polymorphism** refers to minor differences between genes, present in more than 1% of a normal population. For example, eye colour is polymorphic and is determined by different genetic **alleles**.

In the HLA system, there are more alleles. For example, there are over 100 alleles for HLA-A, all of which form a dimer with $\beta_2$-microglobulin. The HLA class II is even more complex; there can be many alleles for the α chain and β chain of each molecule, allowing even more variation. The differences between alleles is very slight but affects whether or not an peptide antigen will bind.

A random sample of individuals will have different HLA genes. Although each individual will be somewhat limited as to which antigenic peptides they can bind and display to T cells, the whole population will express a wide range of HLA molecules and will bind and display many peptides. An individual may not be able to display peptides from a specific infection and may, therefore, not make an immune response (Fig. 3.13.2). However,

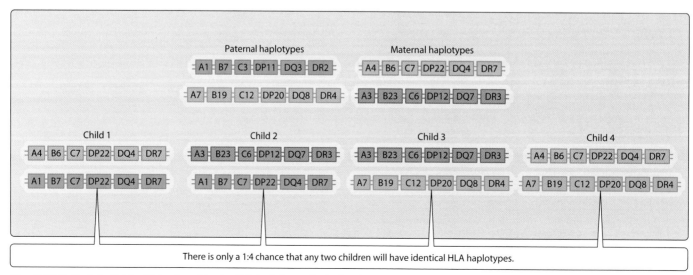

There is only a 1:4 chance that any two children will have identical HLA haplotypes.

**Fig. 3.13.1** Each individual inherits a block of HLA alleles, called a haplotype.

in the population as a whole, at least some individuals will be able to display peptides from the pathogen and develop immunity. This is the molecular basis for the observation that when there is an epidemic of an acute viral infection, some people become quite ill while others develop no symptoms. There are several reasons why dendritic cells are the most effective antigen-presenting cells (Fig. 3.13.3).

Make sure you understand the differences between the genetic mechanisms that enable an *individual* to express many different T cell receptors (through recombination) and a *population* to express many different HLA molecules (through gene duplication and polymorphism).

## RISK OF INFECTION IN HOMOZYGOTES

Individuals who happen to inherit the same HLA alleles from both parents are at higher risk of developing disease from some infections, for example HIV. This is because a heterozygous individual has 12 different HLA alleles, each of which could present an HIV peptide, while a homozygote only has six different alleles. The homozygote has fewer chances of displaying antigen to T cells.

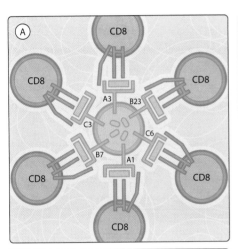

This cell is infected with an intracellular pathogen. It expresses HLA class I molecules, which can present peptide to CD8+ T cells.

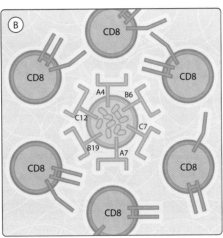

This cell does not have HLA class I molecules able to bind these particular peptides and cannot display to T cells.

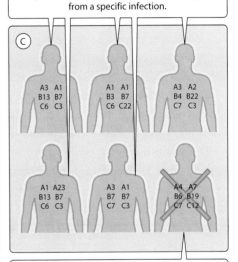

In a random population, most individuals will express HLA molecules able to display antigen from a specific infection.

A few individuals cannot display antigen. In this way, HLA genes affect the risk of disease.

**Fig. 3.13.2** If an individual does not inherit HLA molecules that can bind a particular peptide antigen, they may not respond to a given infection.

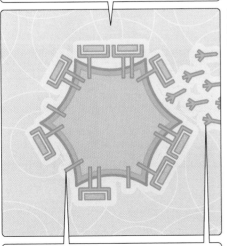

Dendritic cells have a high surface area covered in HLA class I and class II.

Dendritic cells express costimulatory molecules such as CO40 and secrete danger signals such as interleukin-12.

**Fig. 3.13.3** Dendritic cells are the most effective antigen-presenting cells.

# 14. Cytotoxic (CD8⁺) T cells and natural killer cells

## Questions
- Contrast necrosis and apoptosis.
- Describe two mechanisms used by cytotoxic T cells to kill target cells.
- What prevents indiscriminate killing by cytotoxic T cells?
- Describe two ways natural killer cells recognize infected cells.

## HOW CYTOTOXIC T CELLS RECOGNIZE INFECTED CELLS

Interferons are effective at preventing replication of intracellular pathogens (mainly viruses) but do not clear infected cells, which are of little use to the body and best destroyed. This is the role of cytotoxic T cells and natural killer cells.

Cytotoxic T cells are generated in the thymus and express CD8; they recognize cells with specific intracellular infections. Cells containing intracellular infection process antigenic peptides and display them in the groove of HLA class I. The cytotoxic T cell forms an immunological synapse with the infected cell and an activation signal is transmitted. This can lead to killing of the infected cell (Fig. 3.14.1).

Cytotoxic T cells must not kill cells indiscriminately. Their selection in the thymus ensures that CD8⁺ T cells do not recognize normal cells with self-peptides displayed on HLA class I. In addition, cytotoxic T cells will not act unless they receive a danger signal from the innate immune system and 'help' from a special CD4⁺ T cell called a Th1 cell (Chapter 21).

## CELL DEATH

Cells can die two different ways. The first is by **necrosis**, which takes place when cells are damaged by trauma, hypoxia or toxins. During this uncontrolled process the contents of damaged cells are not recycled but leak into the tissues, causing damage.

**Apoptosis** or **programmed cell death** is a more controlled killing process. One result of apoptosis is that the cellular DNA is cut into neat sections by enzymes called **caspases**. This process will also destroy pathogen DNA. Secondly, when a cell dies by apoptosis, its contents form small vesicles wrapped up by the cell membrane. These are phagocytosed by macrophages so their contents are recycled and do not leak out and damage tissues.

Cytotoxic T cells use two processes to induce apoptosis in infected target cells.

- Activated cytotoxic T cells express a molecule called **perforin**, which resembles the membrane attack complex of complement. This punches a hole in the surface of the T cell. An enzyme called **granzyme** is then inserted into the target cell and activates caspases.
- Activated cytotoxic T cells also express a molecule called **FAS ligand**. FAS ligand binds to its partner FAS on the surface of the target cell. FAS has cytoplasmic 'death domains' that activate caspases.

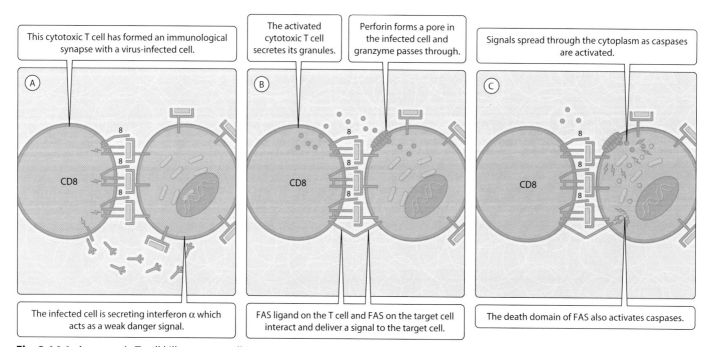

This cytotoxic T cell has formed an immunological synapse with a virus-infected cell.

The activated cytotoxic T cell secretes its granules.

Perforin forms a pore in the infected cell and granzyme passes through.

Signals spread through the cytoplasm as caspases are activated.

The infected cell is secreting interferon α which acts as a weak danger signal.

FAS ligand on the T cell and FAS on the target cell interact and deliver a signal to the target cell.

The death domain of FAS also activates caspases.

**Fig. 3.14.1** A cytotoxic T cell kills a target cell (cont. top page 39).

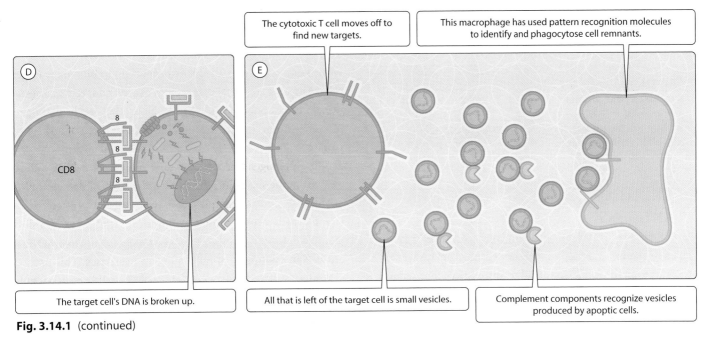

The cytotoxic T cell moves off to find new targets.

This macrophage has used pattern recognition molecules to identify and phagocytose cell remnants.

The target cell's DNA is broken up.

All that is left of the target cell is small vesicles.

Complement components recognize vesicles produced by apoptic cells.

**Fig. 3.14.1** (continued)

## ■ NATURAL KILLER CELLS

Some viruses, particularly members of the herpes family, have evolved ways of evading the immune system. These viruses can prevent cells from expressing HLA class I, blocking recognition by cytotoxic T cells. Natural killer cells have specialized receptors that recognize whether HLA class I is present or not. If HLA class I is absent, natural killer cells go ahead and kill the infected cells, using perforin, granzyme and FAS ligand (Fig. 3.14.2). Natural killer cells can also kill cells that have been coated by antibody, as you will see in Chapter 18.

## APOPTOSIS IN HEALTH AND DISEASE

Apoptosis is used in many parts of the immune system to kill unwanted cells. Cytotoxic T cells and natural killer cells use apoptosis to kill infected cells. Apoptosis is also used in the thymus during T cell development for both positive and negative selection. Similar processes are used in the bone marrow to make sure B cells do not react to self-antigen. There is some evidence that HIV may initiate apoptosis of T cells.

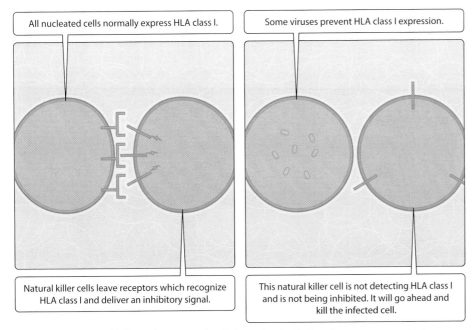

All nucleated cells normally express HLA class I.

Some viruses prevent HLA class I expression.

Natural killer cells leave receptors which recognize HLA class I and deliver an inhibitory signal.

This natural killer cell is not detecting HLA class I and is not being inhibited. It will go ahead and kill the infected cell.

**Fig. 3.14.2** Natural killer cells respond to infected cells that no longer express HLA.

# 15. Macromolecular antigen

## Questions
■ Contrast the antigens involved in cellular and humoral immunity.
■ What are the origins of macromolecular antigens?
■ Explain the terms neutralization, exotoxin and hapten.

## ANTIGENS

Part of the adaptive immune system consists of T cell receptors, which recognize small peptides processed and displayed on HLA. This is sometimes called **cellular immunity**. The adaptive immune system can also use **antibodies** to recognize macromolecular antigens, which do not need to be processed or displayed in any special way; they can be in solution or present on the surface of a pathogen (Fig. 3.15.1). The macromolecules can be peptides, lipids, sugars, nucleic acids, or a mixture of any of these. Immunity mediated by antibodies against macromolecular antigens is sometimes called **humoral immunity**. Antibodies are unable to recognize antigens from intracellular pathogens.

## THE SOURCE OF MACROMOLECULAR ANTIGENS

A variety of structures are present on the surface of organisms. For example, motile organisms use cilia or flagellae to move through liquids. Other organisms use docking molecules to bind onto cells as the first step in infection. For example, influenza virus uses a molecule called haemagglutinin to bind onto target cells. Any of these surface molecules can act as specific antigens for that pathogen (Fig. 3.15.2). Note that each pathogen produces surface molecules that differ from those of any other pathogen.

Some pathogens produce soluble molecules, which diffuse away from the site of infection and cause harm. These are called **exotoxins**. A good example is a toxin produced by *Clostridium tetani*, which causes muscle paralysis, leading to lock-jaw or tetanus. Pathogens tend to produce unique exotoxins, so these are also an example of specific antigens.

Antibody that binds to either surface antigens or soluble exotoxins will prevent infection or prevent the clinical effects of infection, respectively. This is referred to as **neutralization**, which is one of the most useful properties of antibody.

## STRUCTURE OF MACROMOLECULAR ANTIGENS

Macromolecular antigens present abnormal surfaces that are recognized by antibody (Fig. 3.15.3). The surface may be a mixture of substances, for example protein and nucleic acid. The surface may not even be confluent parts of the same molecule, if the molecule is folded. Finally, the antigenic surface may be made up of two entirely different molecules. For example, penicillin is too small to cause an immune response itself but it may link with proteins in red cell membranes. Neither acts as an antigen on its own, but together they become an antigen. In this situation, the penicillin is acting as a **hapten**.

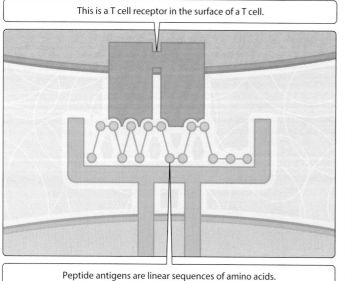

This is a T cell receptor in the surface of a T cell.

Peptide antigens are linear sequences of amino acids.

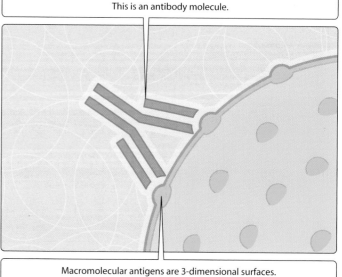

This is an antibody molecule.

Macromolecular antigens are 3-dimensional surfaces.

**Fig. 3.15.1** Antigens recognized by T cells are very different from those recognized by antibodies.

# ■ RECOGNITION BY INNATE AND ADAPTIVE SYSTEMS

You should now be able to distinguish between the molecules recognized by the pattern recognition molecules of the innate immune system and antigen recognition by the adaptive system. The former recognize families of similar molecules produced by a wide range of organisms, for example double-stranded RNA produced by a wide range of viruses. The adaptive immune system recognizes antigens that are usually very specific for one species of pathogen. For example, *C. difficile*, *C. botulinum* and *C. tetani* all produce slightly different exotoxins and thus different antigens. T cell receptors recognize the sequence of amino acids in a peptide antigen. Antibody recognizes the shape of macromolecular antigen. Another name for the adaptive immune system is the **specific immune system**.

## PASSIVE IMMUNITY FOR TETANUS

*Clostridium tetani* spores are found in soil and grow in anaerobic conditions such as dirty wounds, where they produce the exotoxin. To prevent tetanus from developing, patients who have contaminated wounds are given antibodies against tetanus toxin. The antibodies are produced from the blood of donors immune to tetanus. The antibodies *neutralize* the tetanus toxin and prevent tetanus from developing. Using another individual's immunity in this way is referred to as passive immunity.

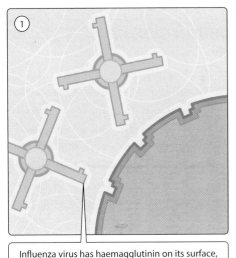

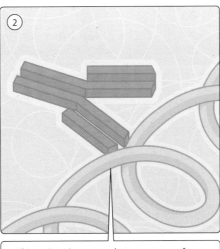

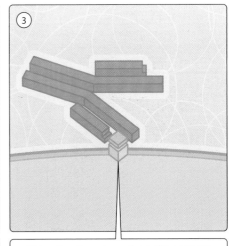

① Influenza virus has haemagglutinin on its surface, which binds onto and attacks cells.

② *Clostridium tetani* bacteria secrete exotoxin.

③ Tetanus toxin binds to neurones and triggers muscle spasm.

**Fig. 3.15.2** Macromolecular antigens are produced by pathogens in a number of ways.

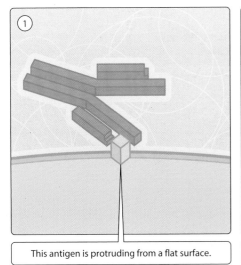

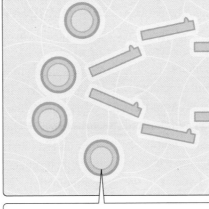

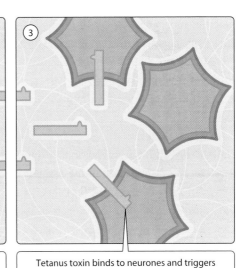

① This antigen is protruding from a flat surface.

② This antigen is a groove between two surfaces. These surfaces are not adjacent in the amino acid sequence of the protein.

③ This antigen is made up of a small exogenous molecule (the hapten) and a larger host protein.

**Fig. 3.15.3** Macromolecular antigens present surfaces to the adaptive immune system.

# 16. Immunoglobulin structure

## Questions
- Contrast the terms antibody and immunoglobulin.
- Explain the following terms: variable domain, Fab fragment, constant region and Fc fragment.
- How is diversity generated in immunoglobulin genes?

## ANTIGEN RECOGNITION BY IMMUNOGLOBULIN LIGHT AND HEAVY CHAINS

The macromolecular antigens described in the previous chapter are recognized by **antibody**. Antibody is made from immunoglobulin molecules. The term antibody is used to describe the functional characteristic, for example the amount of antibody in a blood sample that can bind to tetanus toxin. Immunoglobulin is used to describe the chemical characteristics, for example how many grams per litre of immunoglobulin there are in a blood sample.

Immunoglobulin is a member of the immunoglobulin superfamily and has similar linked domains to HLA and the T cell receptor. In the case of the T cell receptor, peptide antigen is recognized by the $\alpha$ and $\beta$ chains. In the case of immunoglobulin, macromolecular antigen is also recognized by two chains, called heavy and light chains. Variable domains in the heavy and light chains recognize the surface configuration of the antigen. The variable domains form one end of the heavy and light chains, sometimes called the **Fab fragment**, because it is the **f**ragment concerned with **a**ntigen **b**inding. Each immunoglobulin molecule has two Fab fragments and can bind two antigen molecules (Fig. 3.16.1).

The heavy chains, but not the light chains, stretch down to the other end of the molecule. Different heavy chain genes can be used to produce different classes of immunoglobulin. These different classes have various roles, which you will read about in the following chapter. This end of the immunoglobulin molecule is called the **Fc fragment** or constant region.

For the time being we will concentrate on how the variable domains of the light and heavy chains of the Fab fragment are generated.

## IMMUNOGLOBULIN GENE RECOMBINATION

Immunoglobulin is able to recognize specific antigens made up of a very wide range of substances. It is estimated that immunoglobulin must be able to recognize about $10^{11}$ different antigens—T cell receptors only recognize about $10^8$ antigens.

Diversity is increased slightly by having two different light chain genes, $\kappa$ or $\lambda$, either of which can be used to generate immunoglobulin molecules. B cells randomly use either the $\kappa$ or the $\lambda$ light chain genes when they start to undergo genetic recombination.

The $\kappa$ and $\lambda$ light chain genes are both similar to T cell receptor $\alpha$ chain genes. They contain several different $V$ and

**Fig. 3.16.1** The structure of the basic immunoglobulin molecule.

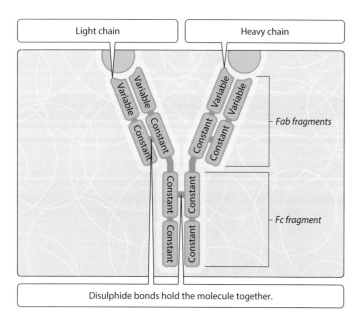

Light chain | Heavy chain

Variable — Variable — Variable — Variable
Constant — Constant — Constant — Constant

Fab fragments

Constant — Constant

Fc fragment

Constant — Constant

Disulphide bonds hold the molecule together.

J gene segments; any two of each are recombined at random to generate the gene for the variable domain. The gene for the immunoglobulin heavy chain is similar to the T cell receptor β gene: it contains *V*, *J* and *D* gene segments, which are recombined at random (Fig. 3.16.2).

Just as for the T cell receptor genes, during recombination of the immunoglobulin genes, DNA cutting by recombinase is imprecise and extra base pairs may be removed and extra base pairs may be added by terminal deoxynucleotide transferase.

## SERUM ELECTROPHORESIS

One way of looking at immunoglobulins is to do electrophoresis. The serum is placed on a gel and an electric charge is placed across the samples. Molecules of different charge and molecular weight move at different rates through the gel. The different plasma proteins are separated into (albumen), α and β regions (acute phase proteins, complement and other proteins) and a γ region. The γ region contains mainly immunoglobulins. Sometimes immunoglobulin is called gammaglobulin. The γ region contains a blur of immunoglobulin of different molecular weights. This reflects the polyclonality of immunoglobulin in the blood. During infections, the total amount of immunoglobulin is increased. This is usually polyclonal (as in the case in Fig. 3.16.3), and it is not possible to see antibodies of different clones.

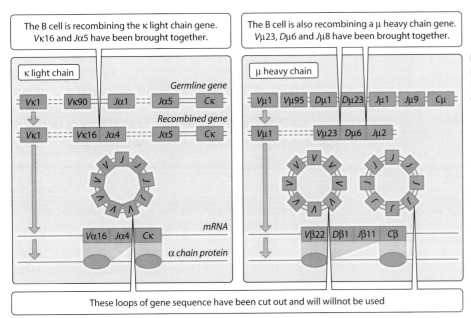

**Fig. 3.16.2** The genetic steps used to produce the variable domains of the immunoglobulin heavy and light chains are very similar to those used to produce T cell receptors.

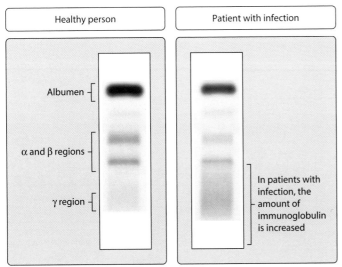

**Fig. 3.16.3** Immunoglobulin molecules produce a blur in the γ region because there are many molecules of differing molecular weight.

# 17. Immunoglobulin classes

### Questions
- How do B cells produce different immunoglobulin classes?
- How do the classes differ in terms of structure, distribution and function?
- What is antibody-dependent cellular cytotoxicity?

## BASIC STRUCTURE

Chapter 16 described how recombination is used to produce many millions of immunoglobulin variable regions at the Fab end of the molecule. Different genetic processes produce the Fc end of the molecules, using constant region gene segments of the heavy chain. There are separate $\alpha$, $\gamma$, $\delta$, $\epsilon$ and $\mu$ constant region gene segments, which are spliced onto the variable region gene segments. These produce immunoglobulin of different **classes**: IgA, IgG, IgD, IgE and IgM (Fig. 3.17.1). Immunoglobulin molecules of different classes may bind the same antigen because they can use the same variable region gene segments.

Immunoglobulin molecules are used in two ways. They can be present as surface molecules, in which case they have a sensor role as the B cell antigen receptor. They can also be secreted and used as effector molecules (Fig. 3.17.2).

Immature B cells initially only produce IgM, but as an immune response develops, they switch to producing other immuno-globulin classes. After class switching, they produce one other immunoglobulin class. To produce immunoglobulin of different classes, the B cell continues to use the same recombined variable region gene segments but switches the heavy chain gene segments encoding the constant region. The differences in the constant region confer the differences between the immunoglobulin classes. Different antibody classes function in different ways.

## IMMUNOGLOBULIN CLASSES

### IgM

IgM is the first antibody to be produced during an immune response. It is present as the B cell receptor on the most immature B cells. The Fc region of IgM enables the molecules to form pentamers, which are effective at neutralizing toxins released from pathogens (Fig. 3.17.3). The lattice of antigen and IgM formed during agglutination is very efficient at activating complement through the classical pathway. This is because complement is most likely to be activated when there are large numbers of Fc regions in close proximity. The large size of the IgM pentamers prevents them from diffusing into the tissues and crossing the placenta.

### IgD

IgD is expressed transiently during B cell development. It is not produced by normal mature B cells.

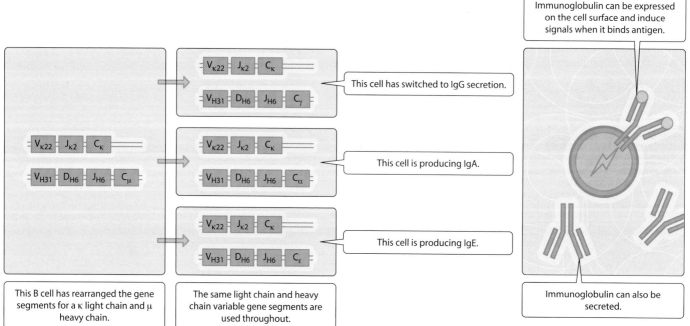

This cell has switched to IgG secretion.

This cell is producing IgA.

This cell is producing IgE.

This B cell has rearranged the gene segments for a κ light chain and μ heavy chain.

The same light chain and heavy chain variable gene segments are used throughout.

**Fig. 3.17.1** Different immunoglobulin classes are produced by switching heavy chain constant region gene segments.

Immunoglobulin can be expressed on the cell surface and induce signals when it binds antigen.

Immunoglobulin can also be secreted.

**Fig. 3.17.2** Immunoglobulin can be expressed as a surface molecule or secreted.

## IgG

IgG is the main antibody secreted into the blood after class switching. The Fc region of the IgG molecule binds well to receptors on cells, for example macrophages. Pathogens coated with IgG are more effectively phagocytosed than uncoated pathogens. This is a type of opsonization and is mediated by receptors for the constant region of IgG. Pathogens coated in complement are also opsonized. Natural killer cells also have Fc receptors, which recognize and kill infected cells. This is called **antibody-dependent cellular cytotoxicity** (as opposed to antibody-dependent complement-mediated cytotoxicity).

## IgA

IgA is also produced later in the immune response. IgA is produced by B cells in mucosal surfaces. The Fc region of IgA enables it to form a dimer and protects it from enzymatic breakdown. This is important because IgA is actively secreted across mucosal surfaces such as the gut.

## IgE

The IgE Fc region binds to specialized Fc receptors on mast cells, even when antigen is absent. If the IgE is cross-linked by antigen (for example a parasitic worm), the mast cell is stimulated to degranulate.

### THE RISK OF INFECTION IN NEWBORN BABIES

Babies that are born prematurely or are not breastfed are at higher risk of infection. This is because they lack passive immunity. Although T cells do not cross the placenta, IgG is actively pumped into the fetus in high quantities during the last few weeks of pregnancy. IgA is present in breast milk and is absorbed intact by babies, giving them some extra passive immunity. These two types of passive immunity protect the newborn baby until it is able to produce antibodies of its own.

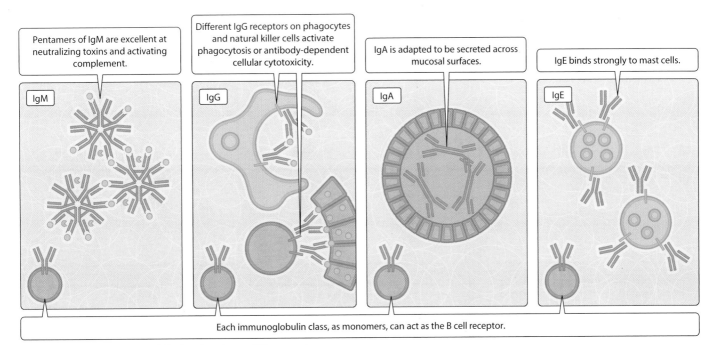

**Fig. 3.17.3** Each immunoglobulin class has a different role.

# 18. B cell maturation and priming

## Questions
- How does negative selection take place in the bone marrow?
- How is B cell self-reactivity prevented in the periphery?
- What is meant by T cell help for B cells?

## B CELL DEVELOPMENT IN THE BONE MARROW

The cells that give rise to both T and B lymphocytes are present in the bone marrow. Pre-T cells migrate to the thymus, while immature B cells mature in the bone marrow.

The first sign of B cell maturation is the recombination of either a κ or a λ light chain gene segment. The IgM heavy chain gene (μ gene) is rearranged next and an intact IgM molecule is expressed on the surface of B cells. This IgM molecule is identical to the IgM that may be secreted as part of the antibody present in blood. IgM attached to the B cell surface forms the B cell receptor.

As is the case in T cells, the B cell receptor is associated with other surface molecules, which are able to transduce signals to the cytoplasm. These signals activate kinases in the cytoplasm and eventually transcription factors migrate to the nucleus, where gene transcription is induced. Although the signalling molecules, transcription factors and genes involved are not the same as in T cells, the principle is similar.

Another similarity with T cell development is that B cell tolerance must be induced (Fig. 3.18.1). In other words, B cells that express a receptor capable of recognizing self-antigen must be killed. Most B cells that recognize a self-antigen in the bone marrow undergo signalling and are killed through apoptosis. This is very similar to negative selection in the thymus. An important difference is that B cells do not recognize antigen in the context of self-HLA, and so a positive selection step is not required.

## B CELL PRIMING

A B cell that has never encountered antigen is described as being naïve. Naïve B cells reside in the lymph nodes, where they encounter antigen from the site of an infected tissue. If the B cell receptor on the surface of a naïve B cell recognizes antigen, a signal is induced, but this is not enough to stimulate antibody production. The B cell also requires **help** from a helper T cell in order to produce antibody.

An activated helper T cell will provide help for the B cell by secreting cytokines such as interleukins 2, 4, 5 and 6. Once the B cell has received these **co-stimulatory signals**, it will start to secrete IgM. A naïve B cell that has been activated in this way is described as being **primed**.

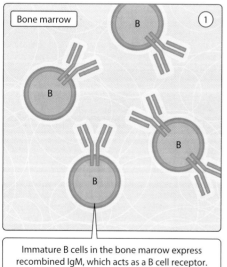

Immature B cells in the bone marrow express recombined IgM, which acts as a B cell receptor.

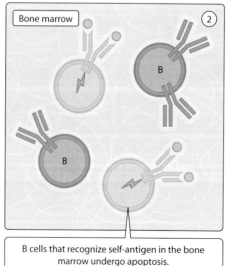

B cells that recognize self-antigen in the bone marrow undergo apoptosis.

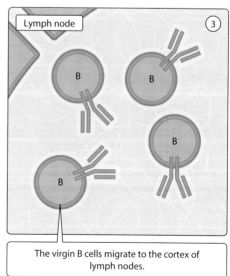

The virgin B cells migrate to the cortex of lymph nodes.

**Fig. 3.18.1** Maturation of B cells and acquisition of tolerrance.

## PERIPHERAL B CELL TOLERANCE

Although most B cells that leave the bone marrow have become tolerant to self-antigen, some escape the negative selection process. To prevent autoimmunity, in other words the recognition of self-antigens, there is a second tolerance step in the periphery. Most B cells require help from helper T cells before they can become fully activated and produce antibody. If a helper T cell and a B cell both recognize antigen derived from a pathogen at the same time and in the same vicinity, the T cell will provide help for the B cell and stimulate it to secrete antibody. This is unlikely to happen with an autoantigen because self-reactive T cells are deleted in the thymus. A B cell that recognizes antigen but does not receive T cell help will become anergic and unable to function.

### X-LINKED AGAMMAGLOBULINAEMIA

BTK is a tyrosine kinase found in B cells and involved in B cell signalling. In X-linked agammaglobulinaemia (antibody deficiency) there is a mutation in the *btk* gene. Boys with this condition have no B cells and produce no antibody (Fig. 3.18.2).

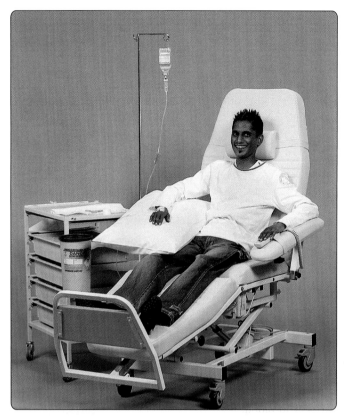

**Fig. 3.18.2** This man has X-linked agammaglobulinaemia. He is having his treatment, intravenous immunoglobulin, which prevents him from getting infection.

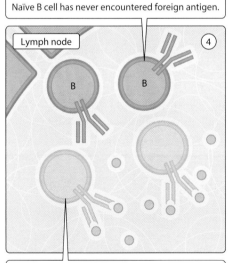

Naïve B cell has never encountered foreign antigen.

Lymph node    ④

B cells reacting to self-antigen and not receiving T cell help become anergic.

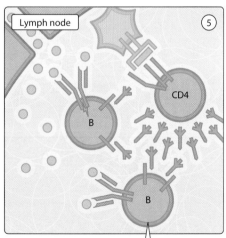

Lymph node    ⑤

CD4

These B cells are recognizing antigen from pathogen *and* receiving T cell help. They are primed.

**Fig. 3.18.1** (continued)

# 19. B cell class switching and hypermutation

## Questions
- How do T cells provide help for class switching?
- What is affinity and how is it affected by somatic hypermutation?
- What is antibody titre?

## IMMUNOGLOBULIN CLASS SWITCHING

IgM is not useful for every situation; for example, IgG is more effective at binding to receptors on macrophages. In addition, IgG has a lower molecular weight than IgM and is able to diffuse into tissues and across the placenta. In order to produce IgG, or other immunoglobulin classes, the B cell undergoes class switching (Fig. 3.19.1). Activated T cells initiate class switching by expressing the surface molecule CD40 ligand, which interacts with a B cell molecule called CD40. Interactions between CD40 and CD40 ligand provides a signal to the B cell to splice a IgG (γ) heavy chain gene segment into the gene. Secretion of IL-4 by the T cell also helps to promote a switch to IgG production.

In the case of a mucosal infection, secretion of IgA would be more useful, which is favoured when the helper T cell secretes IL-4 and TGFβ. Another example is when IgE is required, in which case the T cell secretes IL-4 and IL-13.

In the previous chapter, you learnt how helper T cells are required for B cell priming. Now you also know how helper

T cells are required for immunoglobulin class switching during **secondary responses**. We will return to these important cells in Chapter 21.

## SOMATIC HYPERMUTATION

Different Fab fragments bind to the surface of macromolecular antigen with different strengths. The strength of binding of antibody to macromolecular antigen is referred to as **affinity**.

In order to produce antibody of high affinity, B cells do something very special. Mature B cells that have recognized antigen and started secreting antibody undergo mitosis. During mitosis, mutations are allowed to take place in the gene segments for the immunoglobulin variable domains. **Somatic hypermutation** allows further diversity in the immunoglobulin genes. No other cells in the body permit somatic mutations to take place.

Somatic hypermutation leads to random mutations and most of the time this result in immunoglobulin of lower affinity. B cells that produce antibody of lower affinity will bind antigen less well and will stop receiving stimulatory signals through their B cell receptors. These cells will undergo apoptosis. However, if an antibody of higher affinity is produced, the B cell will continue to be stimulated by antigen (especially if antigen levels are already falling) and so survive to produce more antibody. During an antibody response, the overall affinity of antibody tends to increase. This is called **affinity maturation**.

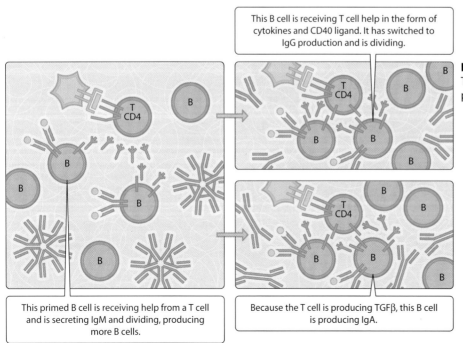

This B cell is receiving T cell help in the form of cytokines and CD40 ligand. It has switched to IgG production and is dividing.

This primed B cell is receiving help from a T cell and is secreting IgM and dividing, producing more B cells.

Because the T cell is producing TGFβ, this B cell is producing IgA.

**Fig. 3.19.1** The type of help provided by T cells dictates the class of antibody produced.

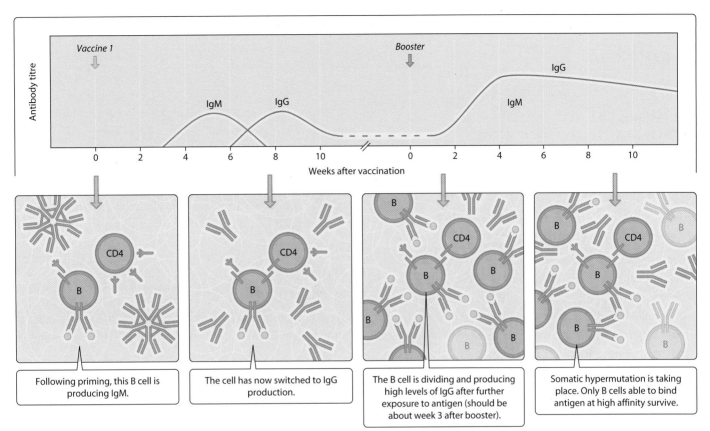

**Fig. 3.19.2** After vaccination or exposure to infection IgM is produced first before a switch to IgG.

The **titre** of an antibody is often used to measure specific antibody; this is the lowest dilution of plasma that can still bind the antigen in the laboratory test. For example, following a vaccination, the titre of antibody to tetanus may increase from 1:5 to 1:1000. The titre is a function of both the physical amount of antibody present and the antibody affinity.

Antibodies initially produced in response to infection tend to fit the antigen rather poorly. They may also, through chance, bind other unrelated antigen. This is referred to as **cross-reactivity**. During somatic hypermutation, affinity for the specific antigen will increase (Fig. 3.19.2). At the same time, peripheral tolerance will tend to ensure that B cells producing cross-reactive antibodies do not survive. So the consequences of somatic hypermutation are that high-affinity, non-cross-reactive (specific) antibodies are produced.

Chapters 12–19 have described the maturation of T and B cells and the interrelating roles of the lymphocyte subsets. Figure 3.19.3 summarizes these subsets. (See also Figs 3.20.1 and 3.21.3.)

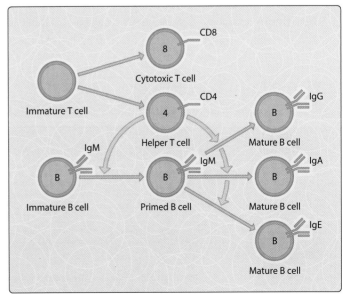

**Fig. 3.19.3** Lymphocyte subsets.

### HYPER-IGM SYNDROME

Some boys are born with mutations in the gene for CD40 ligand, on the X chromosome. This causes a special type of antibody deficiency in which IgM can be produced but other classes of antibody are absent, because class switching cannot take place.

# 20. Plasma cells, memory B cells and T-independent B cells

## Questions
- What are plasma cells and memory B cells?
- Describe three features of a secondary antibody response.
- Describe the special characteristics of T-independent B cells.
- What are the dangers of splenectomy?

## FATE OF ACTIVATED B CELLS

After stimulation by antigen with T cell help, B cells become activated and may undergo class switching and somatic hypermutation. The activated B cells also proliferate, so that many millions of daughter cells produced.

Stimulated B cells can mature into two types of cell: **plasma cells** and **memory B cells** (Fig. 3.20.1). Plasma cells have vast amounts of endoplasmic reticulum and produce large quantities of immunoglobulin. With further help from T cells, plasma cells continue to secrete immunoglobulin until the infection is controlled. A feature of chronic infection is very high levels of polyclonal immunoglobulin in the blood.

Other B cells activated during the primary response mature into memory B cells. Memory B cells are long-lived cells that survive in the germinal centres. If the host is re-exposed to the same pathogen and T cell help is available, these B cells rapidly divide and produce more B cells capable of secreting high levels of IgG, IgA or IgE against the pathogen (Fig. 3.20.2).

High-affinity antibody is a key defence against pathogens because it can neutralize exotoxins, prevent pathogens from entering cells, activate complement through the classical pathway, opsonize pathogens for phagocytosis and stimulate antibody-mediated cellular cytotoxicity. When B memory is present, the immune system can produce a **secondary antibody response** that is rapid and produces high levels of high-affinity specific antibodies. These very useful antibodies can prevent the infection getting a foothold in the host and their production is usually under the control of helper T cells.

## T-INDEPENDENT B CELLS

A minority of B cells do not require help from T cells in order to produce antibody. These T-independent B cells live in special sites such as the spleen and peritoneum, rather than in the lymph nodes. T-independent B cells are stimulated by special kinds of non-protein antigen. Some bacteria, for example *Pneumococcus* and *Haemophilus* spp., have outer capsules containing polysaccharide but no protein, in order to evade phagocytosis, complement and T cells (Fig. 3.20.3). T-independent B cells produce antibodies against these bacteria without T cell help.

T-independent B cells do not recombine their immunoglobulin genes or undergo somatic hypermutation. This means that they produce antibody of low affinity which has a tendency to cross-react with other antigens. For example, antibody driven by sugars present on bacteria can cross-react with sugar antigens on the surface of red blood cells.

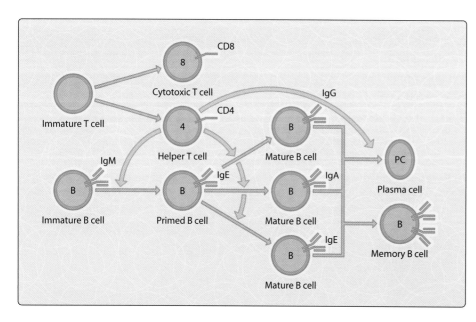

**Fig. 3.20.1** The most highly differentiated B cells—plasma cells and memory B cells—are only produced with help from T cells.

## SPLENECTOMY

The spleen has a major role in preventing infection because it contains a large number of resident phagocytes, which remove opsonized pathogens from the blood. In addition, the spleen is the home to T-independent B cells. Patients involved in accidents sometimes rupture their spleens, which must then be removed. Patients who have undergone splenectomy need antibiotics for the rest of their lives. They are also given vaccines against *Pneumococcus* and *Haemophilus* spp. to boost antibody against these pathogens.

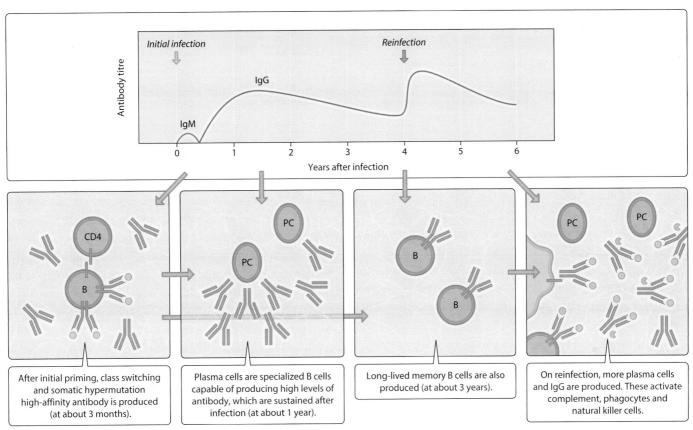

After initial priming, class switching and somatic hypermutation high-affinity antibody is produced (at about 3 months).

Plasma cells are specialized B cells capable of producing high levels of antibody, which are sustained after infection (at about 1 year).

Long-lived memory B cells are also produced (at about 3 years).

On reinfection, more plasma cells and IgG are produced. These activate complement, phagocytes and natural killer cells.

**Fig. 3.20.2** Memory B cells respond to reinfection by producing new plasma cells.

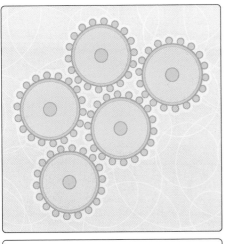

Encapsulated bacteria have large sugar capsules, which do not stimulate T cells or induce conventional antibodies.

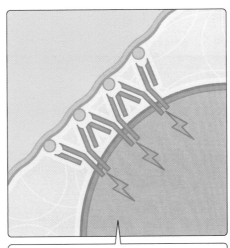

T-independent B cells overcome the need for T cell help by recognizing multiple, repeating sugar motifs.

**Fig. 3.20.3** T-independent B cells are activated by sugar antigens on bacterial capsules.

# 21. T cell memory and T cell help

## Questions
- What are the differences between naïve and memory T cells?
- What are the differences between Th1 and Th2 T cells?
- What are regulatory T cells?

## T CELL PRIMING

CD4+ helper T cells leaving the thymus have never been exposed to the antigen recognized by their specific receptor and are described as **naïve**. Naïve helper T cells are programmed to migrate to the lymph nodes, where they wait to encounter antigen.

Naïve T helper cells respond to antigen that arrives in the lymph nodes on dendritic cells (Fig. 3.21.1). Dendritic cells are present as sentinel cells throughout the body. After they have received a danger signal from interferon α and β, they migrate to the lymph node. Dendritic cells are excellent at presenting antigen to naïve helper T cells.

Once naïve T cells have been activated, they proliferate and become **memory T cells**. Memory T cells have several advantages over naïve T cells:

- there are more memory cells for a specific antigen and they will respond to antigen much faster
- memory T cells are programmed to migrate to the peripheral tissues as well as lymph nodes

- memory T helper cells are specialized to provide help for either cytotoxic T cells or antibody production by B cells.

## DECISION MAKING IN THE IMMUNE SYSTEM

All helper T cells secrete the cytokine IL-2, which stimulates all subsets of lymphocyte (T and B cells and natural killer cells).

Cytotoxic T cells recognize cells infected with intracellular pathogens but will not become fully activated unless they receive help from a helper T cell. These helper T cells secrete interferon γ, which activates cytotoxic T cells, natural killer cells and macrophages. This type of helper response is called a **Th1 response**. Th1 T cells do not 'decide' to promote an attack on intracellular pathogens. The Th1 response is initiated by activated macrophages, which produce the danger signal IL-12 (Fig. 3.21.2).

Th1 responses are not helpful for defending against extracellular pathogens, when antibody production is more useful. The response of a second set of T helper cells, **Th2 cells**, is required for priming B cells and for stimulating immunoglobulin class switching. Th2 cells secrete the cytokines IL-4 and IL-5 to promote B cell maturation and function. It is not yet clear which cells 'decide' to initiate a Th2 response. It may be that an innate cell like a mast cell secretes IL-4 and this initiates the Th2 response.

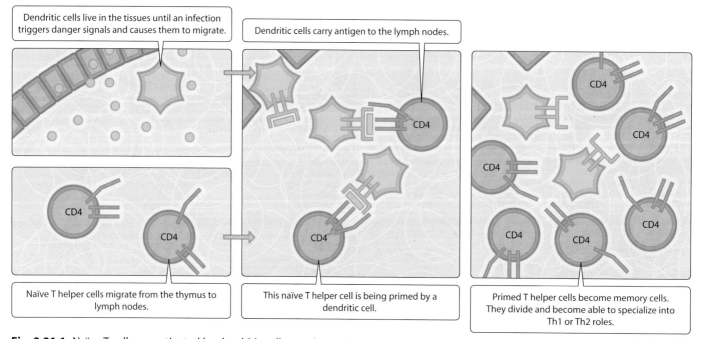

Dendritic cells live in the tissues until an infection triggers danger signals and causes them to migrate.

Dendritic cells carry antigen to the lymph nodes.

Naïve T helper cells migrate from the thymus to lymph nodes.

This naïve T helper cell is being primed by a dendritic cell.

Primed T helper cells become memory cells. They divide and become able to specialize into Th1 or Th2 roles.

**Fig. 3.21.1** Naïve T cells are activated by dendritic cells carrying antigen.

Th1 and Th2 responses promote themselves through positive feedback. Interferon γ secretion by Th1 cells stimulates IL-12 production by macrophages, which promotes more interferon γ secretion. IL-4 secretion by Th2 cells provides positive feedback by encouraging the growth of yet more Th2 cells.

Th1 and Th2 responses inhibit each other through negative feedback: interferon γ secreted by Th1 cells inhibits Th2 cells and IL-4 inhibits Th1 cells.

Initially, most responses to infections are a mixture of varying amounts of Th1 and Th2 response. If infection is not controlled and the response persists, these feedback mechanisms can lead to responses that are very polarized to either Th1 or Th2 cytokines.

A third population of memory T cells appear to switch off the adaptive immune response. **Regulatory T cells** switch off other T cell responses once an infection has been eliminated or when a response against self-antigen has been inadvertently initiated. It is not clear exactly how regulatory T cells 'decide' to do this or how they inhibit other T helper cells.

Figure 3.21.3 summarizes the lymphocyte subsets.

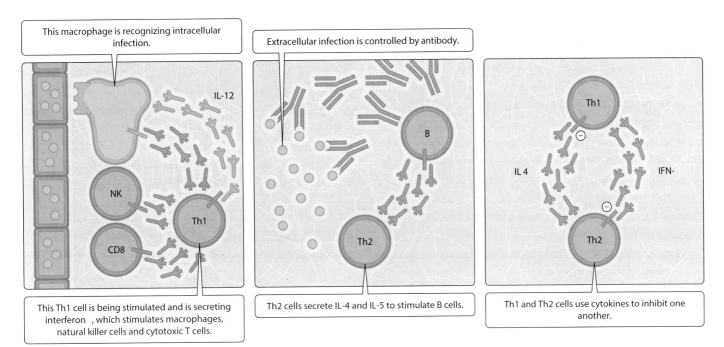

This macrophage is recognizing intracellular infection.

IL-12

This Th1 cell is being stimulated and is secreting interferon  , which stimulates macrophages, natural killer cells and cytotoxic T cells.

Extracellular infection is controlled by antibody.

Th2 cells secrete IL-4 and IL-5 to stimulate B cells.

IL 4        IFN-

Th1 and Th2 cells use cytokines to inhibit one another.

**Fig. 3.21.2** Th1 and Th2 responses.

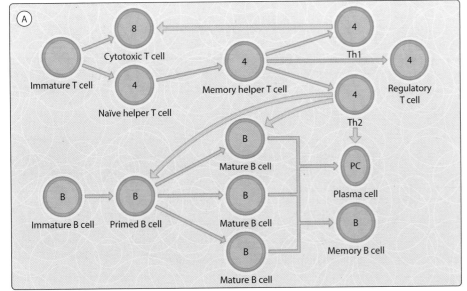

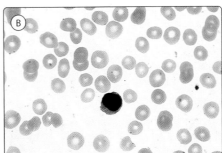

**Fig. 3.21.3** (**A**) All the lymphocyte subsets you are now familiar with. (**B**) a typical lymphocyte. All the lymphocyte subsets (except plasma cells) look very similar using ordinary microscopy.

# 22. The secondary lymphoid organs and mucosa-associated tissues

### Questions
- What are the primary and secondary lymphoid organs?
- What takes place in a germinal centre?
- Name three specialized immunological cells resident in the gut.

## ■ LYMPH NODES

The **primary lymphoid organs**—the **bone marrow** and **thymus**—are the site of production of B and T cells. The **secondary lymphoid organs** are the tissues where T and B cells interact and the adaptive immune system responds to infection. Secondary lymphoid organs include the **lymph nodes**, **spleen** and the **mucosal lymphoid system**. Lymph nodes receive unprimed lymphocytes from blood vessels and antigen and dendritic cells, originating in the tissues, via afferent lymphatics. Antibody and primed lymphocytes produced in the lymph node leave via efferent lymphatics.

Naïve T and B cells are programmed to migrate to the cortex of the lymph nodes. The cortex is an excellent place for lymphocytes to encounter antigen, which enters from the tissues through the lymphatics. Although B cells recognize soluble antigens, T cells respond to antigen presented by dendritic cells migrating from the tissues.

In the cortex, T and B cells and dendritic cells form clusters of interacting cells. The dendritic cells present antigen to T cells, which may provide help for B cells (Fig. 3.22.1).

T and B cells that have been activated by antigen pass from the cortex of the lymph node to form a **germinal centre**. Germinal centres are transient lymph node structures and consist of T and B cells responding to a specific infection. Germinal centres are where B cells undergo class switching and somatic hypermutation and where memory B cells and plasma B cells are produced. Once the infection has been controlled, most of the T and B cells undergo apoptosis and the germinal centres shrink. Some memory T and B cells survive this process in case the antigen is encountered again.

## ■ MUCOSA-ASSOCIATED LYMPHOID SYSTEM

The mucosal surfaces of the gut and respiratory tract have a specialized adaptive immune system. There are many

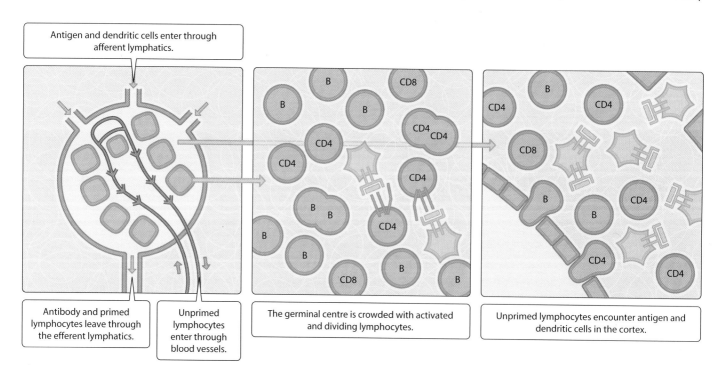

Antigen and dendritic cells enter through afferent lymphatics.

Antibody and primed lymphocytes leave through the efferent lymphatics.

Unprimed lymphocytes enter through blood vessels.

The germinal centre is crowded with activated and dividing lymphocytes.

Unprimed lymphocytes encounter antigen and dendritic cells in the cortex.

**Fig. 3.22.1** Lymph nodes are specialized to promote mixing of T and B cells and for antigen presentation.

similarities with the immune system in other parts of the body, for example there are lymph nodes in the mediastinum that respond to infection in the lung. As well as its role as home for T-independent B cells and splenic macrophages, the spleen acts as a lymph node for the entire gut.

In addition, there is extra lymphoid tissue spread throughout the mucosal surfaces (mucosa-associated lymphoid tissues, MALT). This does not form specialized tissues but occurs in diffuse lymphoid aggregates. In the gut these are known as **Peyer's patches**. **M cells** lie on the surface of the Peyer's patches and are able to pinocytose antigen and present it to underlying T cells. B cells in the gut secrete IgA (Fig. 3.22.2). IgA passes through the cytoplasm of enterocytes, which add a **secretory piece** molecule to prevent enzymatic breakdown.

There are also specialized lymphocytes resident in the epithelium. **Intraepithelial lymphocytes** do not develop in the thymus and use T cell receptors composed of $\gamma\delta$, rather than $\alpha\beta$, chains. Intraepithelial cells secrete inhibitory cytokines, such as **transforming factor $\beta$**. Harmless food antigens absorbed from the gut could stimulate an inappropriate immune response. Intraepithelial lymphocytes act like regulatory T cells and prevent responses to most food antigens.

 **LYMPHADENOPATHY**

A 6-year-old boy has a bacterial infection of his pharynx. His GP notes the reddened pharyngeal mucosa and the raised temperature. The fever is part of an acute-phase reaction. The GP also notes that the lymph nodes in the neck are swollen. Localized lymphadenopathy is part of the normal response to infection but it should resolve when the infection has settled.

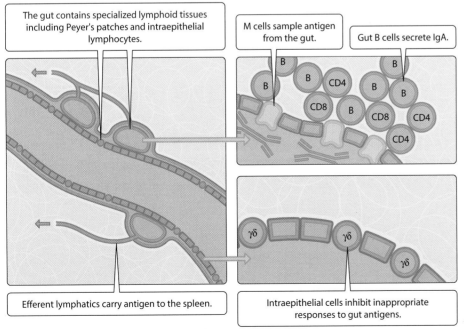

**Fig. 3.22.2** Mucosal lymphoid tissues occur in the gut and respiratory tract.

# 23. Leukocyte migration and trafficking

## Questions
- Describe two of the ligand pairs involved in neutrophil migration. What regulates these molecules?
- How do naïve and memory T cells differ in their trafficking?

## ■ MIGRATION OF WHITE CELLS

Trafficking is the method by which white cells move around the body. This does not happen at random. For example, you already know that:

- macrophages attract neutrophils to the site of extracellular infection
- mast cells attract eosinophils to the site of parasite infection
- during infection, dendritic cells migrate to lymph nodes when they have been stimulated by interferon α or β
- naïve T cell migrate to the lymph nodes, while memory T cells migrate to the lymph nodes and the peripheral tissues.

## Neutrophil movement to infected tissues

Tissue macrophages activated by an infection secrete danger signals such as IL-1 and TNF. These cytokines increase expression of molecules called **selectins** on the lining of local endothelial cells. You will remember that lectins are proteins that bind sugars; selectins bind sugars on the surface of neutrophils. When selectin expression is increased, neutrophils flowing in the bloodstream are slowed and roll along the endothelium. Once the movement of neutrophils has been slowed down, they are stimulated by other danger signals triggered by the infection, for example **chemokines** (produced by macrophages) and **anaphylotoxins** (produced by complement). These signals increase expression of **integrins** on the surface of neutrophils. Integrins bind to intercellular adhesion molecules (ICAMs) on the endothelium. The integrin–ICAM ligand pair forms a much firmer union than selectins and sugars and brings the neutrophils to a complete halt.

Chemokines, anaphylotoxins and arachidonic acid metabolites open up the gaps between endothelial cells. The neutrophils then squeeze into these gaps and enter the tissues. This process is called **diapedesis**. Once in the tissues, the neutrophils follow a trail of chemokines, such as IL-8, secreted by macrophages at the site of infection (Fig. 3.23.1).

## Lymphocyte circulation

Lymphocytes use a trafficking mechanism similar to that described for neutrophils. One difference is that they migrate to specific tissues. Naïve T cells express molecules that form a ligand pair with molecules (**addressins**) on the endothelium in lymph nodes (Fig. 3.23.2). Naïve T cells always leave the blood to enter lymph node cortex, which is exactly where they stand the greatest chance of encountering their antigen.

However, memory T cells home to specific sites in the periphery, where they may come into direct contact with infections. For example, a T cell that originally encountered a

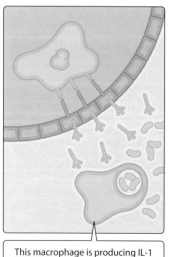

This macrophage is producing IL-1 and TNF, which induce selectin expression on endothelium.

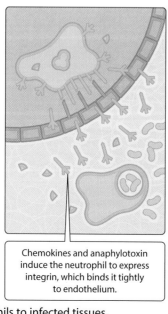

Chemokines and anaphylotoxin induce the neutrophil to express integrin, which binds it tightly to endothelium.

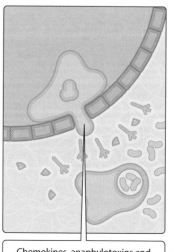

Chemokines, anaphylotoxins and arachidonic acid metabolites open gaps in the endothelium.

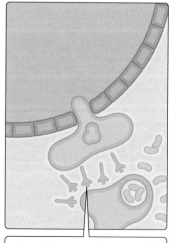

Chemokines attract the neutrophil to the site of the infection.

**Fig. 3.23.1** Migration of neutrophils to infected tissues.

mucosal antigen will express an integrin α4β7. This integrin forms a ligand pair with the adhesion molecule MadCAM1, which is only expressed on blood vessels in the mucosa. The T cell will always return to the mucosa. A T cell exposed to antigen in non-mucosal tissues will express L-selectin, which binds to the adhesion molecule GlyCAM1, expressed on blood vessels in most tissues (but not the mucosa). This T cell will always return to non-mucosal tissues. These ligand pairs ensure that memory T cells always migrate to specific sites. The molecules on the blood vessels (MadCAM1 and GlyCAM1) are called addressins for obvious reasons.

These mechanisms are important because they make sure that white cells only migrate to tissues where they are needed (Table 23.1). If white cells entered tissues at random, it would not just be a waste of white cells, but the cells could cause damage to normal tissues.

## LEUKOCYTE ADHESION DEFICIENCY

Leukocyte adhesion deficiency results from a mutation in the integrin genes. Children with this genetic defect are unable to respond to infection because their leukocytes cannot migrate to the site of infection.

**Table 23.1** LIGAND PAIRS USED IN LEUKOCYTE MIGRATION

| Leukocytes | Endothelium |
|---|---|
| Sugars on neutrophils | Selectins |
| Integrins on neutrophils | ICAM |
| Integrin α4β7 on mucosal memory T cell | MadCAM1: addressin on mucosal tissue |
| L-selectin on non-mucosal memory T cell | GlyCAM1: addressin on non-mucosal tissue |

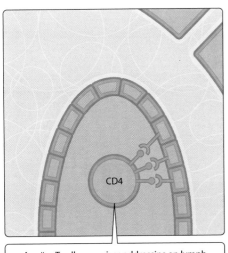

A naïve T cell recognizes addressins on lymph node endothelium.

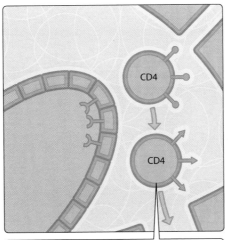

The T cell becomes primed and changes its surface molecules. It leaves via the efferent lymphatics and uses the thoracic duct to reach the blood stream.

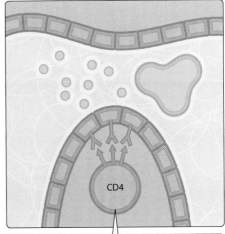

The T cell recognizes addressins on the endothelium in its target tissue.

**Fig. 3.23.2** Migration of lymphocytes.

# 24. Acute inflammation and acute bacterial infection

## Questions
- Give two definitions of inflammation.
- What cells and molecules are involved in triggering inflammation?
- What is septic shock?
- What are the roles of the innate and adaptive immune systems in preventing and clearing acute bacterial infection?

## ■ WHAT IS INFLAMMATION?

Whenever the immune system responds to an infection, there is usually a degree of inflammation. Inflammation is defined clinically as the presence of redness (**erythema**), swelling and pain. Histologically, inflammation is defined as the presence of oedema and white cells in a tissue. Inflammation can be acute, lasting several days, or chronic, usually lasting more than 2 weeks.

The exact type of inflammation depends on the organism that has triggered it. In the next few chapters we will use several common and important infections as examples of the different types of response. The infections we will use are *Staphylococcus aureus* (acute bacterial infection), *Mycobacterium tuberculosis* (chronic bacterial infection) and influenza (acute viral infection).

## ■ ACUTE INFECTION CAUSED BY BACTERIA

Staphylococci are often present in the environment. If the physical barrier of the skin is damaged, for example through a wound, staphylococci start replicating in the tissues. Staphylococci cause local damage at the site of infection.

You already know how the innate immune system responds when a bacterium, such as a staphylococcus, invades the body for the first time (Fig. 3.24.1).

1. Pattern recognition molecules bind onto the bacteria. These activate complement and tissue macrophages, which will start killing bacteria.
2. One of the first changes to occur is increased blood flow (causing erythema) and opening up of gaps between capillary endothelial cells. This causes oedema.
3. IL-1, TNF and chemokines released by macrophages attract neutrophils to the site of infection. These kill the staphylococci and form pus. Staphylococcal infection is sometimes described as **pyogenic**: pus forming.
4. An acute-phase reaction is initiated throughout the body. The most exaggerated form of acute-phase response is **septic shock** (sometimes called systemic inflammatory response syndrome, SIRS). If severe infections trigger production of very high levels of TNF and nitric oxide, the cardiac output and blood vessel tone are decreased, causing very low blood pressure.

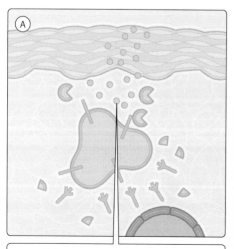

Staphylococci have invaded the skin and are rapidly dividing. A macrophage is activated through Toll-like receptors; complement is also activated.

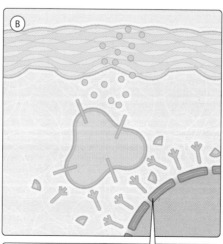

A local blood vessel dilates and endothelium opens up. This causes erythema and swelling.

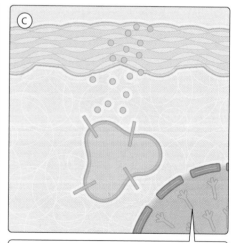

IL-1, IL-6 and TNF enter the bloodstream, triggering an acute phase reaction including fever. GM-CSF increases production of neutrophils in bone marrow.

**Fig. 3.24.1** Acute bacterial infections are mainly cleared by the innate immune system.

Although the abscess formed by the pus can be painful and disabling, these responses are generally enough to eradicate the staphylococcal infection. At the same time as the innate immune system is dealing with the infection, bacterial antigens will pass to the lymph nodes. An early sign of this is swollen local lymph nodes: **lymphadenopathy**. A Th2 response is initiated and anti-staphylococcal antibodies are produced after about 2 weeks. These help to clear the initial infection.

Antibodies may be useful at the end of the infection, but are most important at limiting reinfection. The next time the body is invaded by staphylococci, antibodies will already be present and a memory B cell response will ensure that even more are produced very rapidly. These antibodies help to eliminate the staphylococci more rapidly, by promoting complement activation through the classical pathway and opsonizing the bacteria. Subsequent infections are partially prevented and dealt with by a mixture of innate and Th2 mechanisms.

## BACTERIAL EVASION OF THE INNATE IMMUNE SYSTEM

Several organisms (*Pneumococcus*, *Haemophilus* and *Meningococcus* spp.) have evolved polysaccharide capsules to evade the innate immune system. These capsules are resistant to phagocytosis and the effects of complement. They can cause life-threatening pyogenic infections of the respiratory tract and meninges. Antibodies produced by T-independent B cells protect against these infections but are not produced until late in childhood. Because of their ability to evade the innate immune system, these infections are an important cause of death in children.

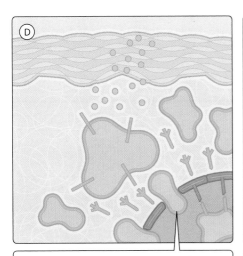

Cytokines, anaphylotoxins and arachidonic acid metabolites attract neutrophils to the site of infection. These form pus.

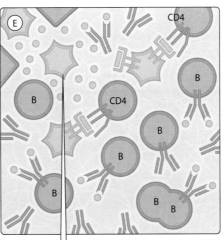

Meanwhile, antigen and dendritic cells reach a local lymph node and stimulate a Th2 response.

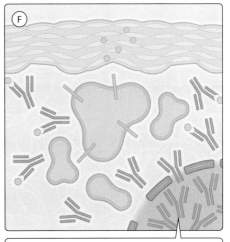

Newly produced antibody clears the infection by activating more complement and opsonizing bacteria.

# 25. Acute viral infection

## Questions
- How are acute viral infections cleared?
- Which parts of the immune system prevent reinfection with specific strains of influenza virus?
- How is influenza virus able to cause reinfection?

### ■ ACUTE INFLUENZA INFECTION

Influenza virus enters the body through the upper respiratory tract. Influenza uses haemagglutinin to bind onto cells. Neutrophils are unable to kill intracellular pathogens like viruses and neutrophil recruitment is not a big feature of viral infections: viruses do not tend to trigger pus formation.

The innate immune system responds to viral infections by producing interferons α and β, which inhibit viral replication and stimulate natural killer cells to destroy the infected cells. Because intracellular pathogens are so inaccessible, these innate measures are only partially effective.

Early in the infection, interferons α and β stimulate dendritic cells loaded with influenza antigens to migrate to the lymph nodes (Fig. 3.25.1). With the help of Th1 cells, specific cytotoxic T cells proliferate and migrate to the site of infection. The T cell proliferation is so dramatic that most of the T cells in the blood during an acute viral infection may have receptors specific for the viral antigens. Cytotoxic T cells are far more effective at killing virus infected cells than natural killer cells. Over several days, all the virally infected cells are killed. This complete clearance of pathogens is called **sterilizing immunity**.

At the same time as cytotoxic T cells are being produced by Th1 response, a Th2 response is also underway. After about 2 weeks, IgM against viral antigens such as haemagglutinin is produced. These antibodies do not help to clear infected cells and have no role in achieving sterilizing immunity.

The role of antibodies is to prevent further rounds of infection of exactly the same strain of virus by producing a rapid **recall response**. IgG produced in a recall response can only act on influenza viruses in the short period between the virus entering the upper respiratory tract and its invasion of cells. IgG binds onto and neutralizes haemagglutinin, thus preventing viruses from anchoring onto target cells. Memory B cells survive in lymph nodes and will protect against exactly the same strain of influenza for many years. IgG can also cross the placenta and protect an unborn child from infection.

During acute viral infections, innate mechanisms are only partially successful and Th1 immunity is required to achieve sterilizing immunity. Th2 immunity helps protect from reinfection later.

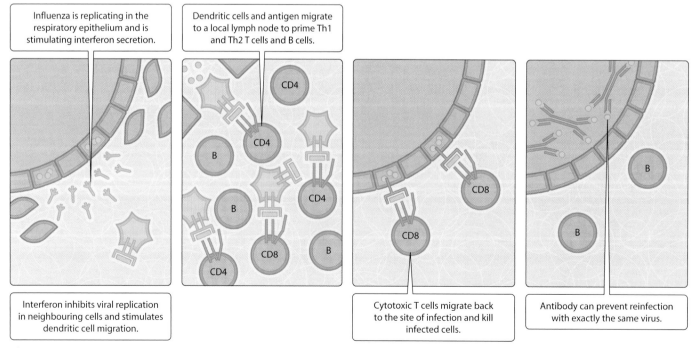

Influenza is replicating in the respiratory epithelium and is stimulating interferon secretion.

Dendritic cells and antigen migrate to a local lymph node to prime Th1 and Th2 T cells and B cells.

Interferon inhibits viral replication in neighbouring cells and stimulates dendritic cell migration.

Cytotoxic T cells migrate back to the site of infection and kill infected cells.

Antibody can prevent reinfection with exactly the same virus.

**Fig. 3.25.1** Response to an acute viral infection.

## Influenza virus epidemics

Influenza is an RNA virus with a small, unstable genome. A characteristic of RNA viruses is that their genomes are prone to mutation. This can occur constantly and slowly through single base pair changes; this is called **antigenic drift**. The influenza genome can also change very dramatically, probably through exchanging genes with animal viruses: so-called **antigenic shift**. This is what can happen when 'bird flu' interacts with human influenza.

Antigenic drift allows slightly different viruses to emerge all the time (Fig. 3.25.2). These viruses may be sufficiently different to escape recognition by IgG antibodies, causing outbreaks of new influenza infection every winter. Antigenic shift results in such major differences in the influenza genome that the virus causes widespread severe infections across entire populations every few years.

### PASSIVE IMMUNITY FOR HEPATITIS B

Hepatitis is a blood-borne infection and can be transmitted to health-care workers after accidents with contaminated needles. This can be prevented with hepatitis B vaccine, which induces IgG against the virus. The IgG prevents the virus from binding to liver cells. If a person who has not been vaccinated has an accident with a contaminated needle, they can be protected from infection by being given immunoglobulin with high titres of antibody against hepatitis B virus.

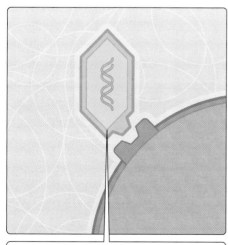
Influenza virus uses haemagglutinin to bind onto target cell.

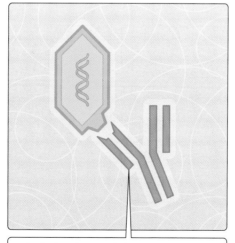
Antibody to haemagglutinin can prevent virus binding target cells; it is a neutralizing antibody.

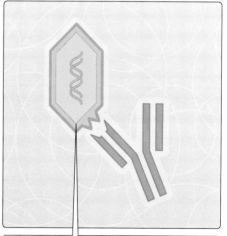
If the virus mutates, the antibody is no longer able to bind and prevent virus binding to target cells.

**Fig. 3.25.2** Antibodies can neutralize viruses, preventing them from infecting cells. Antigenic shift enables viruses to escape neutralization.

# 26. Chronic infection: tuberculosis

## Questions

- How does the immune system control *Mycobacterium tuberculosis* infection?
- Which cells are involved in skin testing for mycobacterial immunity?

*Mycobacterium tuberculosis* (MTB) causes the chronic bacterial infection tuberculosis. MTB enters the body via the lungs and stimulates macrophages by binding onto a specific Toll-like receptor. The mycobacteria are phagocytosed but are resistant to the low pH and enzymes and are capable of staying alive for many years.

Because it is unable to achieve sterilizing immunity, the immune system 'imprisons' the MTB (Fig. 3.26.1). The MTB is held inside the phagosome of long-lived macrophages and the infected macrophages are held inside a **granuloma**. A granuloma is a localized area of chronic inflammation, consisting of specialized macrophages and Th1 cells.

Granuloma formation requires help from Th1 cells. These are primed when dendritic cells migrate to the local lymph node and activate T cells. The Th1 cells migrate to the site of infection and interact with macrophages. Macrophages containing mycobacteria secrete danger signals, such as IL-12, which activate Th1 cells. Mycobacterial antigens presented by macrophages elicit strong specific Th1 cytokine secretion, particularly TNF and interferon γ. These cytokines make macrophages mature into specialist giant cells and epitheloid cells, which are best able to contain MTB. The TNF and interferon γ from Th1 cells stimulate further secretion of IL-12 from the macrophages. A **paracrine loop**—interferon γ from Th1 cells and IL-12 from macrophages—is required to keep the granuloma stable.

Occasionally a small area at the centre of a granuloma becomes necrotic. The necrotic area resembles cheese and this **caseous necrosis** is a hallmark of MTB infection. Calcium may be deposited in the necrotic area and is visible on radiograph.

Initial infection with MTB is called primary tuberculosis and less than 10% of patients have symptoms. Often the only evidence that primary infection has taken place is signs on radiographs of calcification in lungs. However, even with very stable primary lesions, mycobacteria survive for many years. The skin test for mycobacteria is a test for specific immunological memory and for a normally functioning immune system (Fig. 3.26.2).

Post-primary (reactivation) tuberculosis develops in about 10% of infected patients, especially if macrophage or Th1 function is impaired, for example by HIV infection. When this happens, the MTB escape from the granuloma and cause widespread damage throughout the lungs and other parts of the body.

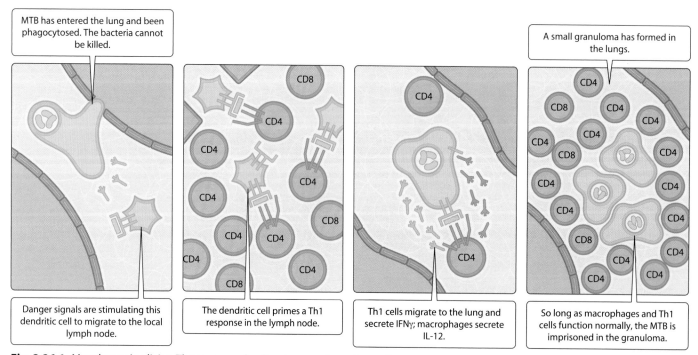

**Fig. 3.26.1** Mycobacteria elicit a Th1 response leading to granuloma formation.

## SKIN TESTING FOR IMMUNITY TO *MYCOBACTERIUM TUBERCULOSIS*

This type of skin test is also known as the Mantoux or Heaf test. In either case, a sterilized mixture of components of MTB are injected intradermally (Fig. 3.26.2). Dendritic cells carry these antigens to lymph nodes and present them to T cells. If the individual has been exposed to mycobacteria before (through infection or vaccination), they will already have very many memory cells specific for mycobacterial antigen. These become activated in the lymph node and subsequently migrate in large numbers to the site of injection. This causes visible inflammation at the injection site after 48 hours (Fig. 3.26.2B). A positive test indicates immunological memory to mycobacterial antigens.

If the individual has never been exposed to mycobacteria before, naïve T cells will be primed following the skin test and a few memory cells will migrate to the injection site. In naïve individuals, there is little sign of inflammation at the injection site, because of the low numbers cells migrating there. A negative skin test can also be seen in a patient who has been exposed to MTB previously but has developed a disorder preventing T cells from functioning normally, such as HIV infection.

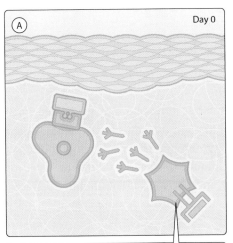

MTB components have been injected into the skin. A danger signal from a macrophage is causing a dendritic cell to migrate to a local lymph node.

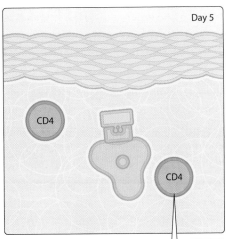

In a previously unexposed patient, very few T cells are available to migrate into the skin. The test is negative.

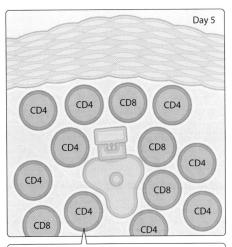

In an exposed patient, there are very many specific T cells able to migrate to the skin. The test is positive.

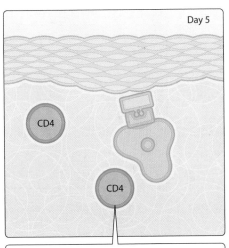

Regardless of previous exposure, patients with defective immune systems are unable to make a response.

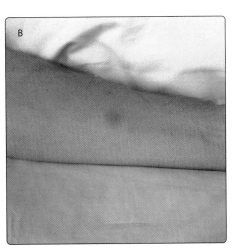

**Fig. 3.26.2** The skin test for mycobacterial infection (**A**) and a positive result (**B**).

# 27. Hypersensitivity

### Questions
- What is hypersensitivity?
- Give examples of hypersensitivity triggered by infection.
- Outline the Gell and Coombs' classification of hypersensitivity.

## ■ HYPERSENSITIVITY TO INFECTIONS

Excessive inflammation caused by the immune system is called hypersensitivity. Hypersensitivity is an important concept in the pathology of many diseases. Sometimes the responses to mycobacterial infection (Chapter 26) can become excessive and may produce large necrotic lesions in the lungs. These can be coughed up, leaving large cavities in the lungs. The damage caused by excessive immune responses also allows mycobacteria to leak from the granuloma and spread from person to person (Fig. 3.27.1A). You learned in Chapter 26 that a poor immune response can lead to post-primary tuberculosis. When the immune response to mycobacteria is excessive, the immune system causes more damage than the pathogen and spreads the pathogen to the next host. The immune response needs to be balanced and regulated in order not to cause damage.

Some chronic viral infections also cause hypersensitivity. For example, hepatitis B virus infects liver cells after passing through the blood. The virus causes very little direct harm to the liver cells. However, there is an excessive immune response to the virus in 10–20% of infected people, which causes on-going liver damage (Fig. 3.27.1B). In these patients with hepatitis B virus infection, excessive Th1 response causes **by-stander damage** to the liver.

It is not clear why some patients have such excessive responses. The likely explanation is that polymorphisms in genes that control the immune response affect whether hypersensitivity can take place in response to these infections.

## ■ HYPERSENSITIVITY TO HARMLESS SUBSTANCES

Harmless environmental substances sometimes cause hypersensitivity. These substances can be any type of molecule, including complicated structures such as proteins or simple molecules like metal ions.

In some individuals, the adaptive immune system recognizes harmless self-antigens that are constituents of normal tissues. This is referred to as **autoimmunity**. Many common diseases are caused by autoimmunity triggering different types of hypersensitivity. These are referred to as **autoimmune diseases**.

All these reactions are reliant on immunological memory mediated by the adaptive immune system. For these reactions to

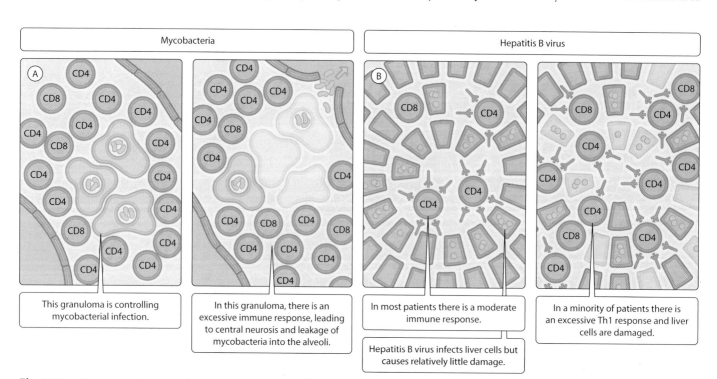

**Fig. 3.27.1** Hypersensitivity to infections: mycobacteria **(A)** and hepatitis B virus **(B)**.

develop, there must be prior exposure to the antigen. Following priming, the effector mechanisms are in place for the hypersensitivity reaction to take place.

## ■ TYPES OF HYPERSENSITIVITY

The **Gell and Coombs'** classification is widely used for hypersensitivity reactions. It is based on the delay between re-exposure to the antigen and the onset of the hypersensitivity reaction (Fig. 3.27.2).

*Type 1: immediate hypersensitivity.* These reactions are triggered when antigen cross-links preformed **IgE** bound to mast cells. There is mast cell degranulation and release of chemical mediators. This causes symptoms within 15 minutes of re-exposure and is referred to as allergy.

*Type 2: antibody-mediated hypersensitivity.* Preformed **IgM** or **IgG** antibodies against cellular components mediate these reactions. The IgM or IgG binds to cells expressing the antigens, and complement or phagocytosis is activated. These reactions can take place within minutes to hours of exposure to the antigen.

*Type 3: immune-complex hypersensitivity.* These reactions also involve **IgM** or **IgG**. In this case, the antibodies form an immune complex with antigen, which activates inflammation. The immune complex can form locally, at the site of antigen re-exposure, or can enter the circulation. Symptoms develop at least 12 hours after re-exposure.

*Type 4: delayed hypersensitivity.* These are Th1-mediated reactions and so involve **Th1 cells** and **macrophages**. T cells must migrate to the site of re-exposure to antigen. Symptoms develop up to 5 days later.

You are now familiar with hypersensitivity to infections. Over the next four sections we describe hypersensitivity to harmless environmental substances. Finally we describe autoimmune diseases: hypersensitivity to self-antigens.

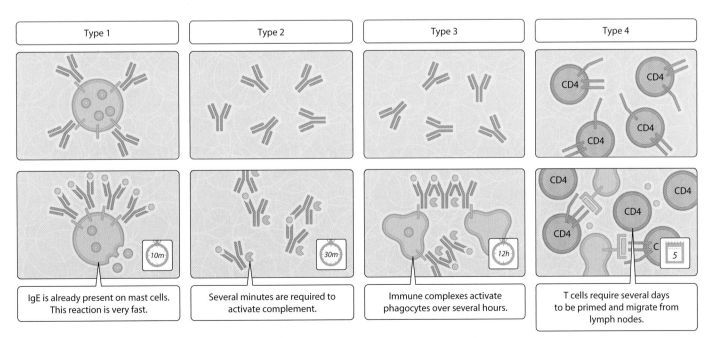

| Type 1 | Type 2 | Type 3 | Type 4 |

IgE is already present on mast cells. This reaction is very fast.

Several minutes are required to activate complement.

Immune complexes activate phagocytes over several hours.

T cells require several days to be primed and migrate from lymph nodes.

**Fig. 3.27.2** Each type of hypersensitivity reaction has a different delay after re-exposure to antigen.

# 28. Immediate hypersensitivity: allergy

### Questions
- Define the following terms; type I immediate hypersensitivity, allergic reactions, allergy, allergen and atopy.
- What happens on the first exposure to an allergen?
- What happens on re-exposure to an allergen?
- What factors affect the risk of allergy?

## SOME IMPORTANT DEFINITIONS

Students sometimes get confused over the terminology used in type 1 hypersensitivity. Make sure you are clear about the following terms:

- **allergy** is the state of having IgE to specific antigens, referred to as **allergens**
- **type I immediate hypersensitivity** is mediated by IgE bound to the surface of mast cells
- **allergic reactions** are clinical symptoms and signs caused through immediate hypersensitivity to specific allergens
- **atopy** is the state of being at high risk of allergies.

Lay people use the term allergy very differently. For example, they may say they are allergic to foods, but this could mean anything from a personal distaste for a food to a pharmacological reaction to chemicals in foods.

## MECHANISMS OF ALLERGY

During the priming response to some antigens in some individuals, there is a marked skewing towards a Th2-type response. In this situation, Th2 cells produce high levels of IL-4 and IL-5, and B cells respond by producing IgE. IgE binds very tightly to specific receptors on mast cells (Fig. 3.28.1).

When the individual is re-exposed to the allergen, the IgE on mast cells is cross-linked. Mast cells respond by releasing their granules and activating arachidonic acid metabolism, in a way similar to how they would respond to a parasitic worm.

Because the IgE is already bound to mast cells and degranulation can occur quickly, the consequences of type 1 hypersensitivity occur within minutes. These immediate effects consist of tissue oedema, mucus secretion and smooth muscle contraction. When the exposure to antigen is localized, for example after inhaling allergenic particles, the effects cause local symptoms such as airways blockage. If the allergen is introduced to the circulation, the effects are much more widespread and there can be catastrophic falls in blood pressure.

If allergen exposure persists, mast cells increase bone marrow production of eosinophils, which migrate to the affected tissue. This causes a second wave of inflammation and damage, which has more lasting effects.

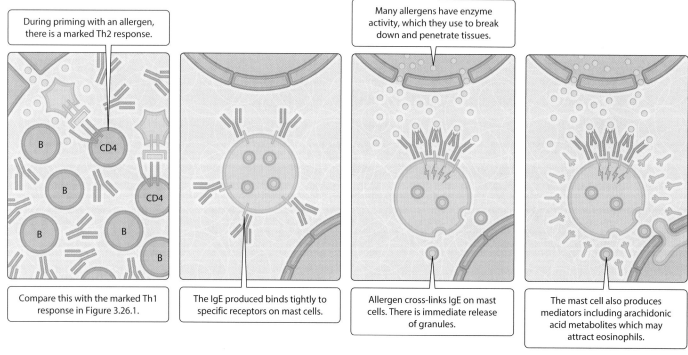

During priming with an allergen, there is a marked Th2 response.

Many allergens have enzyme activity, which they use to break down and penetrate tissues.

Compare this with the marked Th1 response in Figure 3.26.1.

The IgE produced binds tightly to specific receptors on mast cells.

Allergen cross-links IgE on mast cells. There is immediate release of granules.

The mast cell also produces mediators including arachidonic acid metabolites which may attract eosinophils.

**Fig. 3.28.1** After re-exposure to allergen, symptoms develop very rapidly.

Type 1 immediate hypersensitivity involves the innate mechanisms described in Chapter 6 to expel worms. In immediate hypersensitivity, however, IgE is involved and the reactions are driven by harmless substances such as pollens.

## WHY DO PEOPLE GET ALLERGIES?

Allergy is common and its prevalence is increasing. Like most diseases, genetic and environmental factors work together to create a risk of allergy (Fig. 3.28.2).

The genetic factors are not very well understood, but are probably the consequence of inheriting several genetic polymorphisms. For example, the IgE receptor on mast cells (called the FcεR) is polymorphic and inheritance of some alleles may affect the risk of allergy. These polymorphisms are relatively common and up to a third of the population in developed countries are predisposed to allergy (are atopic).

The environmental factors that may be increasing the prevalence of allergy form the basis of the **hygiene hypothesis**. Children brought up on farms or with dogs as pets have a lower risk of developing allergy than those brought up in 'cleaner' environments. It may be that exposure to intracellular pathogens (found in animal faeces) promotes a skewing towards Th1 responses in early life. If this exposure does not take place, the immune response tends to skew towards Th2 responses.

**ATTEMPTS TO REDUCE THE RISK OF ALLERGY**

As you have read, mycobacteria elicit strong Th1 responses. Vaccinating with non-pathogenic *Mycobacterium vaccae* is being used to try and reverse the tendency towards Th2 responses in atopic children.

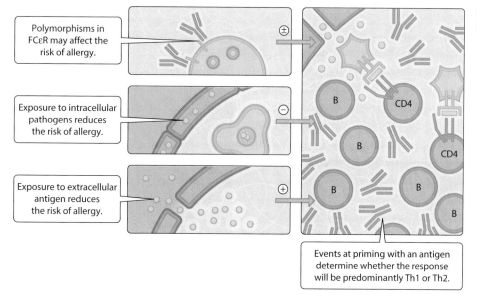

Polymorphisms in FCεR may affect the risk of allergy.

Exposure to intracellular pathogens reduces the risk of allergy.

Exposure to extracellular antigen reduces the risk of allergy.

Events at priming with an antigen determine whether the response will be predominantly Th1 or Th2.

**Fig. 3.28.2** Some of the factors predisposing to allergy.

# 29. Type 1 hypersensitivity: clinical features

**Question**
- Outline the pathological and clinical features of angio-oedema, anaphylaxis, rhinitis and asthma.

## ■ SIGNS AND SYMPTOMS OF ALLERGIES

The signs and symptoms of allergy depend on how the allergen arrives in the body and so which tissues are exposed to allergen.

### Angio-oedema and anaphylaxis

After mast cells have been activated, they release histamine from preformed granules and synthesize prostaglandins and leukotrienes (see Chapter 6). These substances are vasodilators and increase vascular permeability; consequently, an immediate effect is oedema (Fig. 3.29.1). This can be demonstrated in a skin prick test (see below).

If a child with peanut allergy inadvertently eats a small amount of food contaminated with peanut, an immediate consequence can be an attack of **angio-oedema** of the lips or tongue. If the allergen is delivered into the circulation, the effects are much more drastic: for example, when an individual with penicillin allergy is injected with penicillin. Mast cells throughout the body are activated and there is widespread angio-oedema. One effect of this is that swelling can block the upper airways. When large quantities of fluid are shifted from the blood vessels into tissues, the blood pressure can fall dramatically, referred to as **anaphylaxis**.

### Asthma and rhinitis

Air-borne allergens cause symptoms in the nose and bronchi. House dust mite faeces, pollens and animal fur can all do this in allergic people. In these individuals, mast cell activation leads to mucus secretion and smooth muscle contraction, which are consequences of leukotriene synthesis (Fig. 3.29.2).

The exact symptoms depend on the allergen to which a person is sensitized. Allergy to pollens causes nasal symptoms mainly in the summer (seasonal **rhinitis** or **hay fever**), while allergy to house dust mite faeces can cause symptoms all year round (persistent rhinitis). The symptoms are sneezing and runny nose.

If the allergen is small enough to reach the bronchi, it can cause an attack of **asthma**. There is rapid constriction of the bronchi and mucus secretion, causing breathlessness and wheeze. Once the allergen exposure is stopped, these symptoms can rapidly improve, because the bronchoconstriction and mucus secretion are reversible. If exposure continues, eosinophils are attracted to the bronchi. Remember that eosinophils release damaging enzymes, which cause damage to the lungs that is more severe and less reversible.

Atopic individuals often have several different types of allergy. There is also often a family history of allergies in different organs

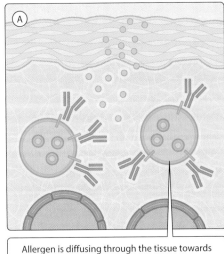
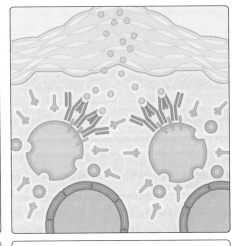
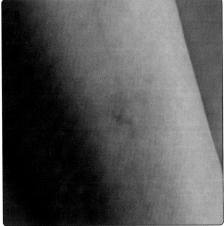

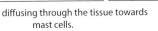
Allergen is diffusing through the tissue towards mast cells.

Histamines, leukotrienes and prostaglandins cause vasodilation and increased vascular permeability. These cause angio-oedema.

**Fig. 3.29.1** **(A)** Angio-oedema occurs rapidly after exposure to allergen. **(B)** This is a typical type 1 immediate hypersensitivity lesion. There is a central oedematous area (the wheal) surrounded by an area of vasodilatation (the flare).

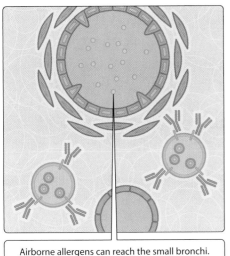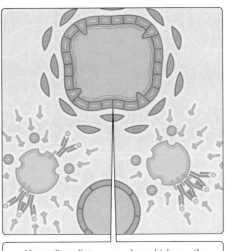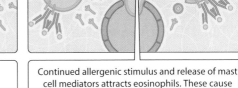

| | | |
|---|---|---|
| Airborne allergens can reach the small bronchi. | Mast cell mediators cause bronchial smooth muscle contraction and mucus secretion. | Continued allergenic stimulus and release of mast cell mediators attracts eosinophils. These cause further damage to respiratory epithelium. |

**Fig. 3.29.2** Damage caused by allergy to air-borne allergens.

and to different allergens, such that a brother may have hay fever and the mother may have year-round asthma.

### Atopic eczema and urticaria

Urticaria is a transient itchy rash consisting of small angio-oedemic lesions. Atopic eczema is a longer-lasting scaly rash. They can both be manifestations of activation of mast cells in the connective tissues in the skin. This can happen after direct contact with an allergen or, particularly in children, can be a manifestation of allergens in foods.

### ■ INVESTIGATING ALLERGY

Skin prick testing is a useful way of confirming that a patient has IgE against a specific allergen (Fig. 3.29.3), but it does not necessarily mean that the allergen was involved in the reaction under investigation; remember that up to a third of the population have IgE to some allergens. Skin prick testing reactions develop in a few minutes. Compare this with the delayed reaction to mycobacterial proteins described in Chapter 26.

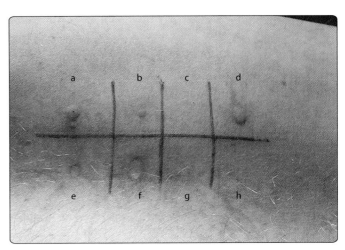

**Fig. 3.29.3** A skin prick test: (a) house dust mite, (b) horse, (c) mould, (d) histamine, (e) guinea pig, (f) dog, (g) cat, (h) saline.

### SKIN PRICK TESTING FOR ALLERGY

Figure 3.29.3 shows a skin prick test used to investigate a man with year-round nasal symptoms. The histamine and saline are positive and negative controls, respectively. He is allergic to house dust mite, guinea pig, horse and dog. Fortunately, he can at least keep his cat.

# 30. Type 2 hypersensitivity: blood group reactions

## Questions
- What is an allogeneic reaction?
- What are the differences between reactions to ABO and to Rhesus antigens?
- What is agglutination and how is it used to test for antibodies?

## BLOOD TRANSFUSION

Red blood cells are often transfused into people who are bleeding or are severely anaemic. They normally behave as a 'harmless environmental substance' but from time to time they can trigger off life-threatening type 2 hypersensitivity reactions. This happens because red blood cells express polymorphic antigens that differ from person to person. Reactions to polymorphic antigens expressed on donor cells are called **allogeneic reactions**. IgM or IgG can bind to these antigens and activate either complement or phagocytosis.

## ABO blood group reactions

There are two alleles for the ABO system, which are expressed co-dominantly. Any individual can express A alone (called A), B alone (B), A plus B (AB) or neither antigen (O). The ABO antigens are sugar molecules and cross-react with bacterial sugar antigens. The bacterial antigens drive the production of antibodies by T-independent B cells (Chapter 20). Previous exposure to allogeneic blood cells is not required to produce antibodies against ABO antigens, and individuals will produce antibodies throughout life to the antigens they do not express. In common with other antibodies produced by T-independent B cells, anti-ABO antibodies are always IgM. For example, an A individual will produce anti-B and an O individual will produce anti-A and anti-B (Fig. 3.30.1).

If a patient is given the wrong blood group, the red cells are immediately bound by IgM. IgM is the most effective antibody at activating complement. The classical complement pathway is activated and the membrane attack complex is rapidly produced and lyses the red cells in the circulation. This is one type of **immune haemolysis**. ABO blood group reactions are a fairly common, avoidable cause of death in hospitals.

## HAEMOLYTIC DISEASE OF THE NEWBORN

Another group of co-dominant red cell antigens form the Rhesus system. Although there are three different antigens (C, D and E), the D antigen is the most important. Most individuals express the D antigen: they are 'Rhesus positive'. The minority of the population do not express the D antigen and are 'Rhesus negative'. The D antigen is a conventional protein antigen and after exposure to D, a Rhesus-negative individual will produce IgG anti-D.

The Rhesus system can cause problems during pregnancy. If a Rhesus-negative mother has a child to a Rhesus-positive father, the fetus is likely to express D. During the first pregnancy, some

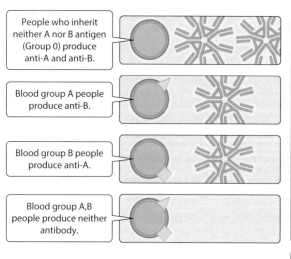

People who inherit neither A nor B antigen (Group 0) produce anti-A and anti-B.

Blood group A people produce anti-B.

Blood group B people produce anti-A.

Blood group A,B people produce neither antibody.

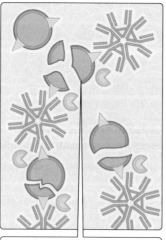

If, for example, group A cells are transfused into a B donor, IgM rapidly binds the cells, activates complement and destroys the cells.

**Fig. 3.30.1** Mechanism of ABO blood group reactions.

fetal red cells may leak across into the maternal circulation, priming her to make antibodies. These antibodies are unlikely to reach a significant titre during the first pregnancy.

If she has a second pregnancy with a Rhesus-positive fetus, IgG anti-D antibodies can cross the placenta and reach the fetal circulation. IgG is not very good at activating complement and the fetal red cells are not destroyed in the circulation. Instead, the red cells become opsonized and are phagocytosed in the fetal spleen (Fig. 3.30.2). This causes a gradual onset, but very severe, anaemia in the fetus.

Note that anti-ABO antibodies are IgM. IgM does not cross the placenta and so does not tend to cause problems during pregnancy.

## AGGLUTINATION

Antibodies are able to clump together—**agglutinate**—particles expressing appropriate antigens. Agglutination can be used to test for antibodies (Fig. 3.30.3). A Rhesus-negative woman without antibodies will not be able to agglutinate Rhesus-positive red cells. If she has a sufficient titre of anti-D, her serum will be able to agglutinate Rhesus-positive cells. This type of test is referred to as a **Coombs' test**. Note that complement is not present in this test or the cells would be rapidly lysed.

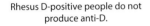
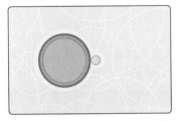

Rhesus D-positive people do not produce anti-D.

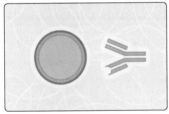

Rhesus D-negative people produce anti-D after exposure.

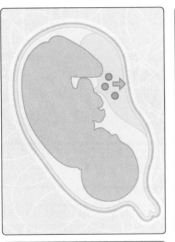

During pregnancy with a Rhesus D-positive fetus, red cells may leak into the mother.

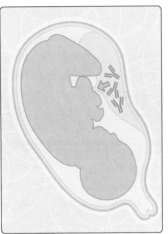

In a subsequent pregnancy with a Rhesus D-positive fetus, IgG is produced and crosses the placenta into the fetus.

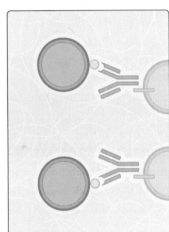

IgG is not good at activating complement but opsonizes red cells, which are destroyed in the fetal spleen.

**Fig. 3.30.2** Haemolytic disease of the newborn occurs in a rhesus D-positive fetus carried by a Rhesus D-negative woman.

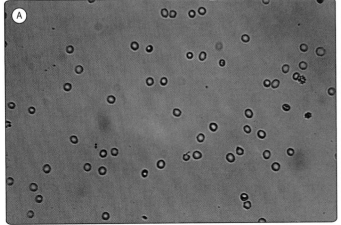
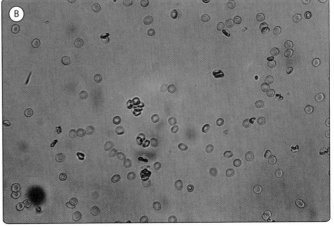

**Fig. 3.30.3** Red cell agglutination induced by a serum sample. **(A)** No agglutination **(B)** Agglutination.

# 31. Type 3 hypersensitivity: immune-complex disease

**Questions**
- What are immune complexes?
- Describe how localized and circulating immune complexes cause different symptoms.

## ▪ IMMUNE COMPLEXES

In the previous section, you learnt how antibodies can agglutinate antigens present on the surface of particles. Antibodies are also capable reacting with soluble antigen and forming lattices of antibody and antigen, referred to as immune complexes. Small immune complexes are soluble. Larger immune complexes—which tend to form when antigen and antibody are present in equimolar quantities—may be insoluble.

Immune complexes are part of the physiological response to infection. For example, when a pathogen is producing high quantities of an exotoxin and the host is responding with high titres of antibody, immune complexes may form.

Immune complexes often form during infection. Because they contain large numbers of Fc regions in close proximity, immune complexes are excellent at activating the classical pathway of complement cascade (Fig. 3.31.1). Even IgG activates complement efficiently when it forms immune complexes.

Because they can cause harm, the immune system has a mechanism for clearing complexes. The immune complexes and complement bind to complement receptors on red cells. The red cells transport the complexes to the spleen, where they are removed harmlessly by phagocytes. The phagocytes in the spleen are macrophages which engulf immune complexes without producing a danger signal. However, if complexes form rapidly at a local site or if they overwhelm these systems, they can trigger inflammation. This kind of inflammation is the cause of type 3 hypersensitivity.

## ▪ LOCAL IMMUNE-COMPLEX DISEASE

Sometimes immune complexes form in response to harmless environmental antigens. For example, people who work in air-conditioned buildings sometimes inhale large quantities of mould spores. These can trigger high titres of IgG antibodies. The mould spores and IgG interact in the lung, forming immune complexes. These immune complexes form so quickly that they cannot be removed by red cells. Anaphylotoxin produced by the reaction attracts neutrophils, triggering inflammation (Fig. 3.31.2). The patient will develop difficulty breathing, usually several hours after exposure to the spores: so-called humidifier lung. This is a type of hypersensitivity because the spores are not harmful in their own right.

Note that mould spores can also trigger immediate hypersensitivity in the form of asthma. This also causes difficulty in breathing. The two different problems can easily be distinguished by the timing of the symptoms after exposure to the mould:

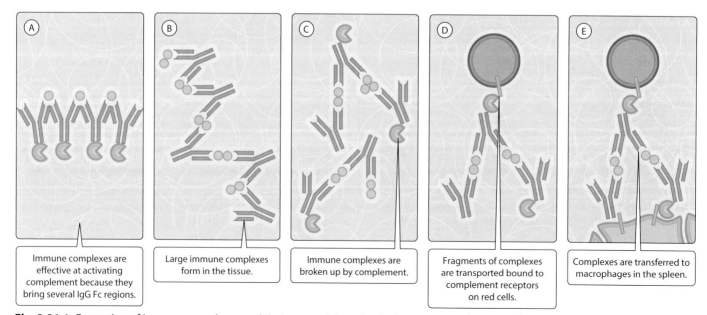

**Fig. 3.31.1** Formation of immune complexes and their removal by red cells. Immune complexes can form in tissues or in solution in the blood.

mould-induced asthma happens immediately after exposure to mould spores, while humidifier lung symptoms develop several hours after exposure. Also, patients with immediate hypersensitivity will have a positive skin test after skin prick testing with mould spores.

## ■ CIRCULATING IMMUNE COMPLEXES

In other situations, large quantities of immune complex form and enter the circulation. This can happen when large quantities of antigen are injected, for example with some drugs, such as penicillin.

On re-exposure to the drug, immune complexes form in the bloodstream. **Circulating immune complexes** can trigger acute inflammation but tend to do so in specific parts of the body, usually the joints, skin and kidneys (Fig. 3.31.3). For reasons that are not well understood, circulating immune complexes produced elsewhere in the body are deposited in these tissues. Typically, a patient will develop joint pains, rashes and kidney problems several days into a course of penicillin injections.

### IMMUNE-COMPLEX DISEASE IN INFECTIONS

Infections that cannot be cleared sometimes lead to high-level production of IgG. The IgG can combine with antigens from pathogens and immune complexes then form. This can happen with hepatitis virus infection and malaria. Kidney problems commonly occur as a result of deposition of these immune complexes.

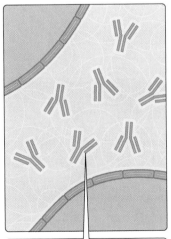

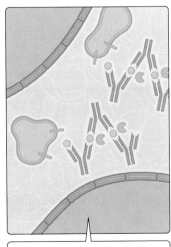

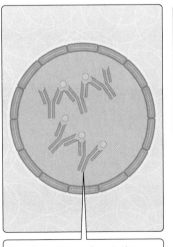

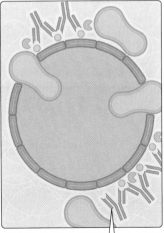

| | | | |
|---|---|---|---|
| Previous exposure to mould spores has induced antibodies in the lung tissues. | When more spores are inhaled, immune complexes form. These activate complement, which attracts neutrophils to the lung. | Immune complexes in the circulation have overwhelmed the clearance mechanism. | Complexes deposit below the basement membrane, activating complement and recruiting neutrophils. |

**Fig. 3.31.2** For humidifier lung to develop, there must be preformed anti-mould antibodies in the lung tissue.

**Fig. 3.31.3** Circulating immune complexes tend to be deposited in blood vessels in the skin, kidneys and joints.

# 32. Type 4: delayed hypersensitivity

## Questions
- What is delayed hypersensitivity?
- Which cells are involved in contact dermatitis?
- Using reactions to penicillin as an example, describe the different types of hypersensitivity.

## CONTACT DERMATITIS

In Chapter 26 you learnt how some chronic infections with pathogens lead to inflammation dominated by T cells and macrophages. The macrophages secrete IL-12 and the Th1 cells secrete interferon γ. These reactions always take several days to develop. Once they have developed, IL-12 and interferon γ maintain sites of chronic inflammation until the antigen is cleared. For example, inflammation appears several days after the antigen has been applied in skin testing for *Mycobacterium tuberculosis*. This type of response is useful when it is controlling mycobacterial infection, but when it takes place in response to harmless environmental antigens it can cause damage and is referred to as **delayed hypersensitivity**.

Harmless environmental substances can trigger delayed hypersensitivity. A good example is contact dermatitis, where inflammation occurs at the site of contact with the allergen. The most common antigen is nickel, and very often the inflam-mation appears under jewellery or clothes fastenings.

The nickel is able to enter the outer layers of the dermis, where it combines with normal host proteins (Fig. 3.32.1). Neither nickel on its own nor the host protein is able to act as an antigen, but nickel behaves as a **hapten** (Chapter 15). Haptens become antigenic after they combine with host proteins. The nickel–protein complex is taken to the lymph nodes by dendritic cells and Th1 T cells are recruited. The next time the patient's skin is exposed to nickel, these specific T memory cells migrate to the affected site and secrete interferon γ. The inflammatory response then develops over several days.

Sometimes, it is not easy to determine the exact antigen in contact dermatitis, for example in a patient exposed to many different chemicals at work. In patch testing, several candidate chemicals are applied to the skin and covered with a dressing (Fig. 3.32.2). After 48–72 hours, the skin is examined. Inflammation develops under the antigen that is causing the symptoms. In this case, the patient has reacted to three separate chemicals he is exposed to at work.

## MIXED HYPERSENSITIVITY REACTIONS

The Gell and Coombs' classification is an idealized scheme. Some hypersensitivity reactions contain elements of more than one type of reaction. For example, acute asthma after exposure

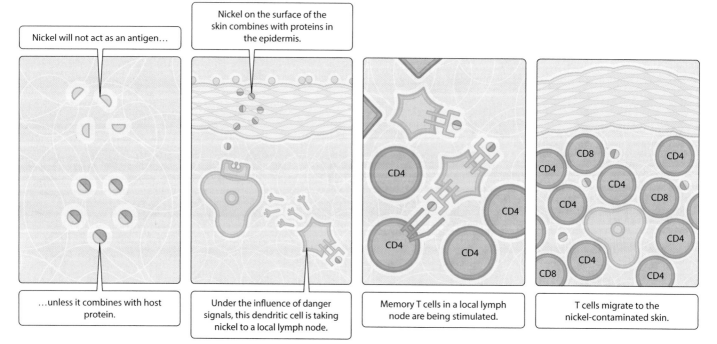

| Nickel will not act as an antigen… | Nickel on the surface of the skin combines with proteins in the epidermis. | | |
|---|---|---|---|
| …unless it combines with host protein. | Under the influence of danger signals, this dendritic cell is taking nickel to a local lymph node. | Memory T cells in a local lymph node are being stimulated. | T cells migrate to the nickel-contaminated skin. |

**Fig. 3.32.1** Contact dermatitis caused by re-exposure to an allergen.

to an antigen such as cat fur has all the characteristics of type 1 immediate hypersensitivity. If exposure to the antigen persists, eosinophils are attracted to the airways and more chronic inflammation then develops. The reaction then develops some features of a type 4 reaction, with production of Th1 cytokines, although there is no granuloma formation.

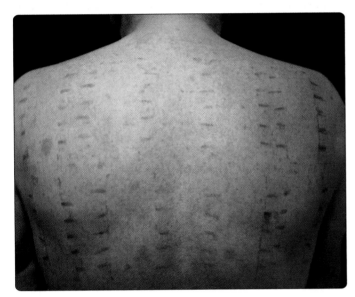

**Fig. 3.32.2** Patch testing.

## DRUG HYPERSENSITIVITY

Drugs are 'harmless environmental substances' but, from time to time, they can cause hypersensitivity reactions. Penicillin is a good example of a drug that produces different types of reaction (Fig. 3.32.3). If patients produce IgE against penicillin, allergies can occur immediately after exposure. Penicillin is quite a common cause of fatal anaphylaxis. Penicillin can also bind onto red blood cells and act as a hapten. If an individual makes IgG or IgM antibodies against penicillin, the red cells can be destroyed within hours, resulting in haemolysis. Penicillin can also cause immune-complex disease when IgG antibodies are produced. The symptoms of joint pain and kidney problems develop over several days. Penicillin can cause delayed hypersensitivity reactions. For example, if penicillin ointment is used, contact dermatitis can develop several days later.

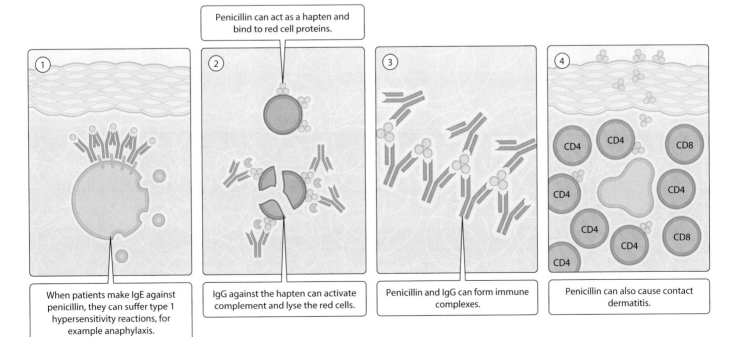

Penicillin can act as a hapten and bind to red cell proteins.

1 — When patients make IgE against penicillin, they can suffer type 1 hypersensitivity reactions, for example anaphylaxis.

2 — IgG against the hapten can activate complement and lyse the red cells.

3 — Penicillin and IgG can form immune complexes.

4 — Penicillin can also cause contact dermatitis.

**Fig. 3.32.3** Any of the four different hypersensitivity reaction mechanisms can cause reactions to penicillin. How would the timing of the reactions differ in each case?

# 33. Autoimmunity

## Questions
- How do autoantibodies occur?
- Which two genetic factors lead to the breakdown of thymic tolerance?
- Which environmental factor may lead to breakdown of peripheral tolerance?

## ■ WHAT IS AUTOIMMUNITY?

When antibodies and T cells recognize normal components of the body, autoimmunity is said to be present. Autoimmune responses can sometimes, but not always, lead to disease, which we describe over the next four sections. **Autoimmune disease** is mediated by hypersensitivity reactions types 2, 3 and 4. First of all, you need to understand how autoimmunity occurs in normal people.

The T-independent B cells described in Chapter 20 do not require T cell help and so can produce antibodies that cross-react with normal self-antigens. These autoantibodies are produced at low levels and do not have very high affinity. Autoantibodies against, for example, single-stranded DNA are present in many normal people, particularly the elderly, and do not necessarily cause disease.

For autoimmune disease to develop, tolerance to self-antigen must break down at two levels: in the thymus and in the periphery.

## How thymic tolerance breaks down

Type 1 diabetes is a good example of an autoimmune disease and is caused by autoimmune destruction of pancreatic islet cells. Normally, T cells that react to islet cell antigen plus HLA in the thymus undergo apoptosis during negative selection (Fig. 3.33.1). This process can fail in two ways.

- The individual may have inherited, through chance, an HLA allele that does not strongly bind the self-antigen. For example, an individual who inherits the HLA allele DQ2 has a high risk of developing type 1 diabetes, probably because this allele does not present islet cell antigens (e.g. insulin) well and so autoreactive T cells cannot be deleted.
- For negative selection to be effective, the thymus must be able to display a wide range of the body's normal peptide antigens. For example, insulin is normally expressed and displayed in the thymus. If an individual inherits gene polymorphisms that reduce the thymic expression of insulin, there is a risk that T cells that recognize insulin will not be deleted.

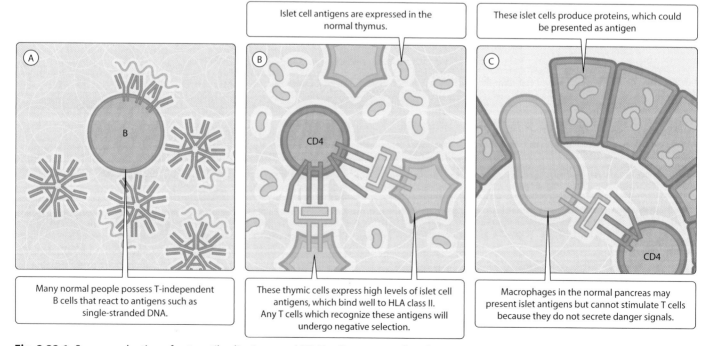

**Fig. 3.33.1** Some production of autoantibodies is normal (**A**). T cells are normally tolerized to antigen in the thymus (**B**) and periphery (**C**).

Inheritance of *DQ2* and a poorly active insulin promoter can prevent thymic tolerance to islet cell antigens. If one or both of these genetic factors are present, self-reactive T cells may escape to the periphery (Fig. 3.33.2). Not everyone with these genetic risk factors will develop type 1 diabetes, because peripheral tolerance must break down before disease can develop.

## How peripheral tolerance breaks down

Even after binding to antigen plus HLA, T cells will not react unless they receive a danger signal. Self-reactive T cells may reach the pancreatic islet and recognize antigen; however, unless they receive a danger signal, they will become anergic (Chapter 12).

The likely factor to trigger a danger signal in type 1 diabetes is infection, which could lead to the innate immune system secreting cytokines such TNF or IL-1. These danger signals would increase lymphocyte migration into the organ and then stimulate self-reactive T cell responses. Although, at the moment, there is no direct evidence that infection acts in this way, the concept that genes and environment work together to break down tolerance is probably correct.

### SUSCEPTIBILITY TO AUTOIMMUNE DISEASE

Because genetic factors predispose to autoimmune disease, an individual with one disease is likely to develop another. For example, patients often have both type 1 diabetes and autoimmune thyroid disease. Autoimmune diseases also tend to run in families.

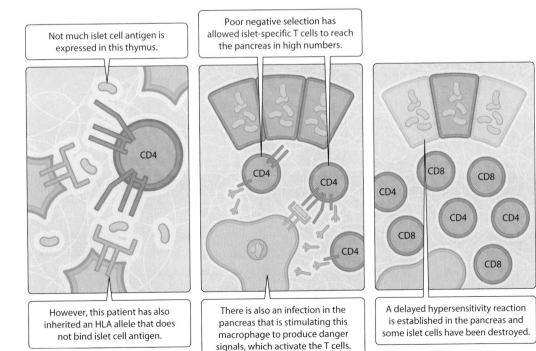

Not much islet cell antigen is expressed in this thymus.

Poor negative selection has allowed islet-specific T cells to reach the pancreas in high numbers.

However, this patient has also inherited an HLA allele that does not bind islet cell antigen.

There is also an infection in the pancreas that is stimulating this macrophage to produce danger signals, which activate the T cells.

A delayed hypersensitivity reaction is established in the pancreas and some islet cells have been destroyed.

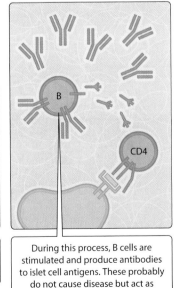

During this process, B cells are stimulated and produce antibodies to islet cell antigens. These probably do not cause disease but act as markers of type I diabetes.

**Fig. 3.33.2** Several genetic and environmental factors need to be in place for autoimmune diseases like type 1 diabetes to develop.

# 34. Antibody-mediated autoimmune disease

### Questions
- Outline the pathology of autoimmune haemolytic anaemia, Goodpasture's syndrome, Graves' disease and Wegener's granulomatosis.
- How is direct immunofluorescence carried out?

Although autoantibodies can be harmless, they can also bind to cells and cause damage through type 1 hypersensitivity. In a slight variation, autoantibodies binding to cells can also directly affect cell function.

### ■ AUTOIMMUNE CELL DESTRUCTION

Chapter 29 described how transfused or fetal red blood cells can be destroyed in part of a response to allogeneic antigen. Drugs such as penicillin can sometimes trigger haemolysis, if the patient makes anti-penicillin antibodies.

Normal host red blood cells can also sometimes be attacked by autoantibodies, causing **autoimmune haemolytic anaemia**. In this situation, antibodies are reacting to normal red cell antigens. The clinical features and speed of red cell destruction depend on the type of antibody present. IgM autoantibodies are good at activating complement and so haemolysis takes place

| (A) Red blood cells |
|---|

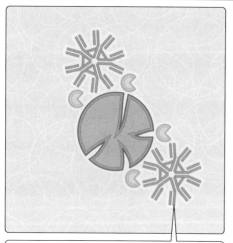 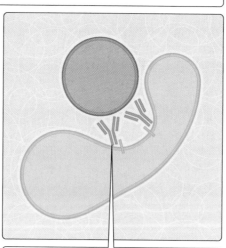

**Fig. 3.34.1** Autoimmune damage: (**A**) red cell destruction; (**B**) damage to soft tissues.

IgM anti-red cell antibodies cause rapid haemolysis by activating complement.

IgG anti-red cell antibodies cause more gradual destruction by macrophages in the spleen.

| (B) Solid tissues |
|---|

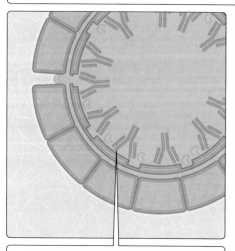 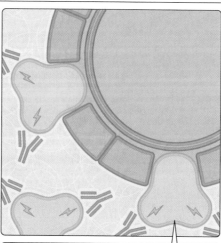 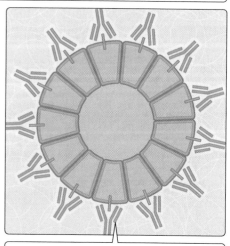

In Goodpasture's disease, IgG damages basement membrane in the kidney.

In Wegener's granulomatosis, IgG binds to neurophils in the kidneys. These become activated and cause tissue damage.

In Graves' disease, IgG binds to the TSH receptor, stimulating thyroid activity.

very rapidly in the circulation. IgG autoantibodies, by comparison, tend to opsonize red cells, which are gradually destroyed in the spleen (Fig. 3.34.1a).

Autoantibodies can sometimes also damage platelets and neutrophils.

## AUTOIMMUNE EFFECTS ON CELL FUNCTION

Autoantibodies can also damage solid tissues. In **Goodpasture's syndrome**, IgG autoantibodies are produced against the basement membrane in the glomerulus and lungs. The IgG antibody binds onto the basement membrane and activates an inflammatory response (Fig. 3.34.1b).

IgG autoantibodies can also stimulate excessive cell function. In **Wegener's granulomatosis** there are autoantibodies against neutrophil cytoplasmic proteins. These antibodies activate neutrophils, which then undergo respiratory burst and release their proteolytic enzymes. Wegener's granulomatosis also causes tissue damage in the lungs and kidneys.

A second and commoner type of stimulatory antibody is found **Graves' disease**, which is caused by autoantibodies against the thyroxin-stimulating hormone (TSH) receptor on thyroid epithelium cells. When the IgG binds, it mimics the effects of TSH, causing growth of thyroid cells and increased secretion of thyroxine. This causes enlargement of the thyroid and hyperthyroidism.

Autoimmune diseases caused by antibody binding to cells all have very different clinical features, depending on the tissues involved. They do have some features in common, however.

- If a piece of tissue can easily be obtained, the IgG antibody can be found deposited at the site of tissue damage, using a technique called **direct immunofluorescence** (Fig. 3.34.2).
- If a patient is pregnant, the IgG autoantibodies may cross the placenta and cause the disease in the fetus.
- The disease can be treated by removing the antibody. **Plasmapheresis** is a rather complicated procedure in which blood is taken from the patient and the patient's plasma is separated and removed. More often it is simpler to use immunosuppressive drugs targeted at reducing B cell function.

### DIRECT IMMUNOFLUORESCENCE IN GOOD PASTURE'S DISEASE

If tissue can be obtained from an affected patient, direct immunofluorescence can be used to show where antibody has bound in vivo (Fig. 3.34.2). A tissue section is prepared and incubated with antibody produced in an animal against IgG (anti-IgG). The anti-IgG is linked to a fluorescent chemical, which emits bright visible light when activated by invisible ultraviolet light. After incubation, unbound anti-IgG is washed away. When the tissue is viewed under a microscope and illuminated with ultraviolet light, the anti-IgG will fluoresce. In Goodpasture's disease, IgG can be seen bound to the glomerular basement membrane. There is little fluorescence in the neighbouring renal tubules.

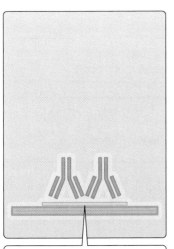

A tissue biopsy section is placed on a glass slide. It contains the patient's IgG already complexed to the tissue in vivo.

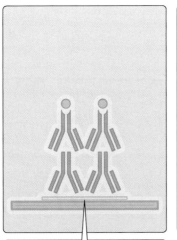

The tissue is incubated with anti-IgG linked to a fluorescent molecule.

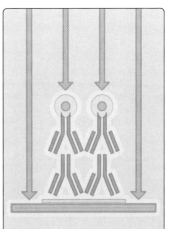

When it is viewed with ultraviolet light, the fluorescent molecule gives off visible light.

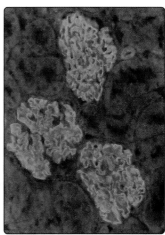

This is a direct immunofluorescence view of a kidney biopsy from a patient with Goodpasture's disease. There is IgG along the basement membrane.

**Fig. 3.34.2** Direct immunofluorescence.

# 35. Systemic lupus erythematosus and tests for autoimmunity

### Questions
- Which organs are affected by SLE?
- Which processes normally prevent DNA antibodies from being made?
- What are the connective tissue diseases?
- Describe two methods for detecting autoantibodies present in blood samples.

## ■ SYSTEMIC LUPUS ERYTHEMATOSUS (SLE)

SLE is an autoimmune disease caused by circulating immune complexes: type 3 hypersensitivity. The main antigen in the immune complexes is double-stranded DNA and the antibodies are IgG anti-DNA. There are also autoantibodies against ribonucleoproteins—nuclear proteins associated with DNA—called Ro, La, Sm and RNP and against other cellular components.

In circulating immune-complex disease, there tends to be damage to the joints, skin and kidneys. This is the case in SLE, in which patients develop joint inflammation (arthritis), a facial rash, made worse by exposure to ultraviolet, and progressive renal damage (Fig. 3.35.1). The IgG antibodies can also cross the placenta and cause damage to the fetus in pregnant women with SLE.

IgM antibodies against single-stranded DNA are produced in low levels in some healthy people and do not seem to cause disease. B cells are not normally exposed to double-stranded DNA because when cells die through apoptosis the DNA is held in vesicles that are rapidly phagocytosed (see Chapter 14). Any DNA that does leak out of cells activates complement and mannose-binding lectin, becomes opsonized and is also rapidly phagocytosed. In these ways, DNA is normally rapidly sequestered (hidden) by the innate immune system. The adaptive immune system does not normally encounter double-stranded DNA and does not become tolerant to it. SLE is more common in patients with defects in apoptosis, complement and mannose-binding lectin: when these clearance mechanisms fail, B cells recognize double-stranded DNA and start producing IgG antibodies.

SLE is one of several autoimmune conditions known as the **connective tissue diseases**, each of which is linked to antibodies against different nuclear components (Fig. 3.35.2). Each connective tissue disease affects different organ systems, usually including the skin, joints and kidneys, although immune complexes are not implicated in each case.

### Diagnosis of SLE

SLE can be confirmed by finding autoantibodies against double-stranded DNA. Two different types of test can be used to show

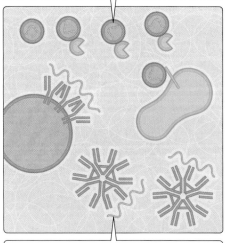

DNA from apoptotic cells is usually cleared by the innate immune system.

IgM antibodies against single-stranded DNA are present in some normal people.

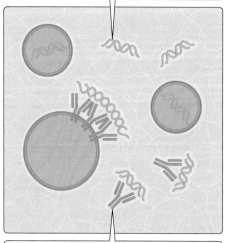

When innate systems fail, the adaptive immune system is exposed to double-stranded DNA.

B cells may then produce IgG antibodies against double-stranded DNA.

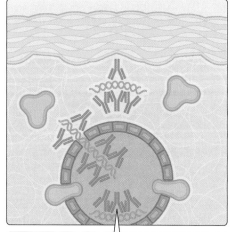

IgG–DNA complexes are formed in the tissues, circulation and trigger inflammation.

**Fig. 3.35.1** Systemic lupus erythematosus.

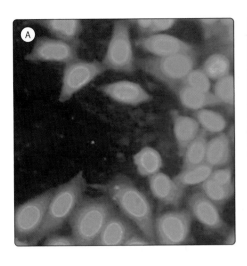
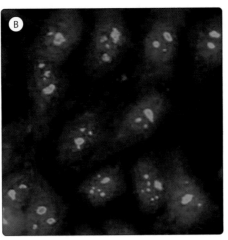

**Fig. 3.35.2** Indirect immunofluorescence is used to detect antinuclear antibodies in the connective tissue diseases. in SLE, the antibodies against DNA 'light-up' the entire nucleus (**A**). In the related disease, system sclerosis, the antibodies are directed against the nucleolus only (**B**).

anti-DNA antibodies. The first is **indirect immunofluorescence (IIF)** for **anti-nuclear antibodies**. This test is very similar to direct immunofluorescence (described in Chapter 34). In IIF the patient's serum is incubated with a glass slide covered in a layer of cells. Antibodies present in the serum will bind onto the nuclei of the immobilized cells (Fig. 3.35.2). Fluorescent anti-IgG is then added and the procedure continues as in the direct method. Anti-nuclear antibodies are produced at low titre by quite a few normal people and people with infections. These antibodies are against a mixture of nuclear antigens not necessarily just DNA, so their presence does not always confirm a diagnosis of SLE. In other words, anti-nuclear antibodies are not a specific test for SLE.

A more specific test for anti-DNA antibodies is an enzyme-linked immunosorbent assay—better known as ELISA (Fig. 3.35.3). Purified DNA is used as the antigen in ELISA tests; any IgG detected will be specific for DNA. ELISA tests thus give more specific results for SLE than indirect immunofluorescence for anti-nuclear antibody.

ELISA tests are used to measure antibodies in a very wide range of settings, not just autoimmunity. For example, they can be used to measure antibodies to specific pathogens to check whether an infection has taken place or whether a vaccination has been successful.

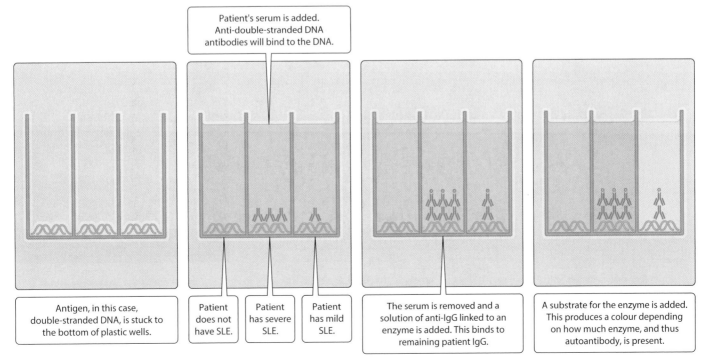

Patient's serum is added. Anti-double-stranded DNA antibodies will bind to the DNA.

Antigen, in this case, double-stranded DNA, is stuck to the bottom of plastic wells.

Patient does not have SLE.

Patient has severe SLE.

Patient has mild SLE.

The serum is removed and a solution of anti-IgG linked to an enzyme is added. This binds to remaining patient IgG.

A substrate for the enzyme is added. This produces a colour depending on how much enzyme, and thus autoantibody, is present.

**Fig. 3.35.3** Detection of autoantibodies by enzyme-linked immunosorbent assay (ELISA).

# 36. Rheumatoid arthritis

## Questions
- What are the clinical features of rheumatoid arthritis?
- What are the effects of TNF in rheumatoid arthritis?
- What is rheumatoid factor?
- Compare corticosteroids and TNF-blocking drugs in the treatment of rheumatoid arthritis.

## ■ CLINICAL FEATURES

Rheumatoid arthritis is common and leads to severe disability by causing chronic inflammation in the synovial membranes of joints. The inflammation affects joints symmetrically and, although it often initially affects the small joints of the hand, it can affect any synovial joint in the body. In early disease, rheumatoid arthritis causes inflammation in synovium, which is swollen to a hundred times its normal size, causing pain and stiffness. As the disease progresses, the bone near the joints is destroyed and inflammation spreads along the synovium of tendon sheaths. These changes destroy joints and related tissues and cause irreversible disability.

## ■ PATHOLOGY

In rheumatoid arthritis, there is a delayed (type 4) hypersensitivity reaction in the synovium. The autoantigen that drives this process is still not known, but Th1 cells and macrophages invade the synovium. Tumour necrosis factor (TNF) is secreted by both of these cell types and causes much of the damage. TNF has the following effects (Fig. 3.36.1):

- it increases leukocyte adhesion to endothelium and is chemotactic: more leukocytes are attracted to the synovium
- it acts as a danger signal for T cells and activates macrophage, acting as positive feedback for inflammation
- it stimulates osteoclasts (which are derived from macrophages) to destroy bone
- it mediates an acute-phase response, and the C-reactive protein and the erythrocyte sedimentation rate (indicating blood viscosity) are increased; the term 'acute' phase is not very appropriate here because the course of the disease tends to run for years.

Rheumatoid arthritis also stimulates B cells to produce autoantibodies in about 70% of patients. The characteristic autoantibody is an IgM antibody against IgG and is referred to as **rheumatoid factor**. There are popular misconceptions about rheumatoid factor. The first is that it causes the joint problems—this is not the case. The second is that it is a diagnostic test for rheumatoid arthritis. This is incorrect because rheumatoid factor is not present in all patients. In addition, like very many autoantibodies, rheumatoid factor is often present in the blood of patients with infection. Rheumatoid factor is neither sensitive nor specific for rheumatoid arthritis.

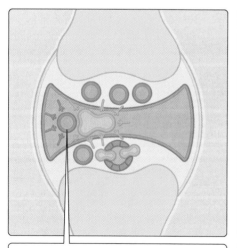

In early rheumatoid arthritis, T cells and macrophages interact to produce TNF and recruit more cells to joints.

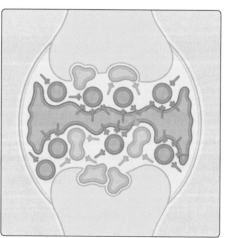

In advanced rheumatoid arthritis, there is considerable synovial swelling and some bone destruction.

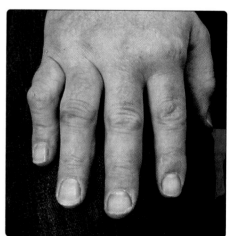

This patient's hand shows characteristic swelling of the small joints.

**Fig. 3.36.1** TNF causes much of the inflammation and joint deformity in rheumatoid arthritis.

# TREATMENT: ANTI-INFLAMMATORY DRUGS

Anti-inflammatory drugs are very often used to treat autoimmune diseases, including rheumatoid arthritis. Many different anti-inflammatory drugs have been used over the years (Fig. 3.36.2). Aspirin and other non-steroidal anti-inflammatory drugs (NSAIDs) prevent pain and the production of the arachidonic acid metabolites such as prostaglandins. They have some joint-protecting properties.

Traditionally, corticosteroids have often been used. Corticosteroids act mainly on macrophages and other antigen-presenting cells, in which they inhibit synthesis of over 100 proteins. In common with all drugs which inhibit the immune system, corticosteroids increase the risk of infections. In addition, they have effects on many other tissues and frequently cause side effects such as high blood pressure, bone thinning and psychiatric problems. Newer drugs of choice for rheumatoid arthritis are rapidly replacing corticosteroids. Infliximab is a monoclonal antibody against TNFα.

## TNF-BLOCKING DRUGS IN RHEUMATOID ARTHRITIS

In recent years, TNF-blocking drugs have been introduced. These drugs, for example infliximab, are recombinant proteins that bind to TNF and prevent it from interacting with TNF receptors. These drugs rapidly switch off the symptoms of rheumatoid arthritis and are more effective and safer than corticosteroids. Like all other immunosuppressive drugs, they do increase the risk of infection. However, in the case of TNF-blocking drugs, this appears to be mainly an increased risk of tuberculosis (Chapter 26), emphasizing the special role of TNF in combating this infection.

In rheumatoid arthritis, inflammatory mediators are produced by macrophages and T cells.

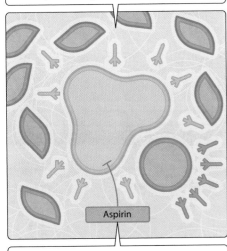

Aspirin

Aspirin and other NSAIDs inhibit synthesis of prostaglandins and reduce pain.

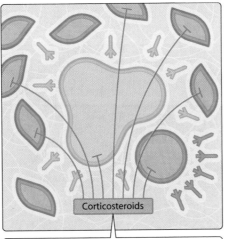

Corticosteroids

Corticosteroids inhibit synthesis of proteins in many different cells. They are very effective but cause many side effects.

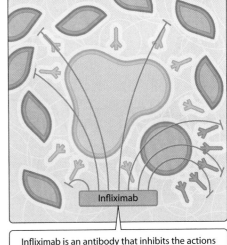

Infliximab

Infliximab is an antibody that inhibits the actions of TNF and prevents damage to joints.

**Fig. 3.36.2** Drugs for rheumatoid arthritis vary in their effectiveness and side effects.

# 37. Lymphoid malignancies

## Questions
- What is meant by monoclonality?
- How does chromosomal translocation cause lymphoid malignancy?
- Which viral infections cause lymphoid malignancy?

## MALIGNANCY OF THE ADAPTIVE IMMUNE SYSTEM

Here, we deal with malignancies that arise from the cells of the adaptive immune system, which are sometimes referred to as **lymphoid malignancies**. This topic does not cover malignancies that arise from cells of the innate immune system, such as precursors of neutrophils, usually referred to as **myeloid malignancies**.

The normal immune response is **polyclonal**: at any one time the immune system contains immunoglobulin and T cell receptors that are a mixture of millions of different specificities. Occasionally, for example at the peak of a response to an infection, the immune response becomes **oligoclonal** and there are very few different immunoglobulin or T cell receptors detectable. These represent the immunoglobulin or T cell receptors that are specific for the antigens produced by the infection.

**Monoclonality** refers to the situation when there is only a single immunoglobulin or T cell receptor detectable (Fig. 3.37.1). This situation usually occurs when a single B or T cell has become immortalized and retains the ability to proliferate, giving rise to millions of progeny cells. These squeeze out the normal polyclonal response. Each of these cells has undergone identical T cell receptor or immunoglobulin gene rearrangement.

## HOW LYMPHOID TUMOURS ARISE

Lymphoid malignancies are relatively common. Like most malignancies, they can occur because an oncogene has become permanently switched on, forcing the cell to divide continuously. In lymphocytes, a second mechanism can come into play. Lymphocytes are prone to apoptosis and after a normal immune response to an infection, most T and B cells will undergo apoptosis and die. If this process is interfered with, the cells can survive indefinitely. Genetic defects which damage the apoptosis mechanism can also immortalize cells.

Two types of process can switch on oncogenes or prevent apoptosis in lymphocytes (Fig. 3.37.2). The first process is chromosomal **translocation**, which happens when there are chromosomal breaks that are not properly corrected. This can incorrectly align an oncogene with a promoter for another gene. If the promoter is permanently activated, for example an immunoglobulin or T cell receptor promoter, the oncogene will also become permanently switched on. This can force cell cycling or give protection from apoptosis. T and B cells are particularly prone to translocation because they use genetic recombination to generate their receptor genes. During recombination, the wrong genes may be joined together (Fig. 3.37.2).

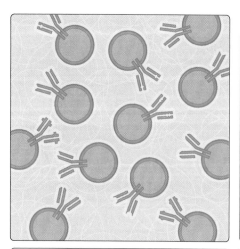
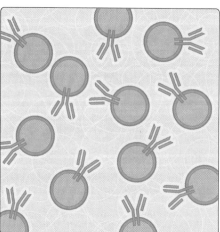
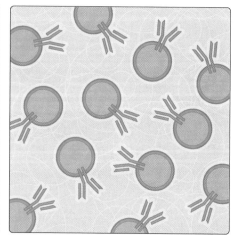

The normal resting immune system is polyclonal; each B or T cell has a different receptor.

In response to some infections, the immune system may become oligoclonal: only a handful of different receptors are expressed.

A monoclonal immune system is always abnormal and usually reflects malignancy. An identical receptor is expressed on each cell.

**Fig. 3.37.1** The clonality of the immune system reflects health.

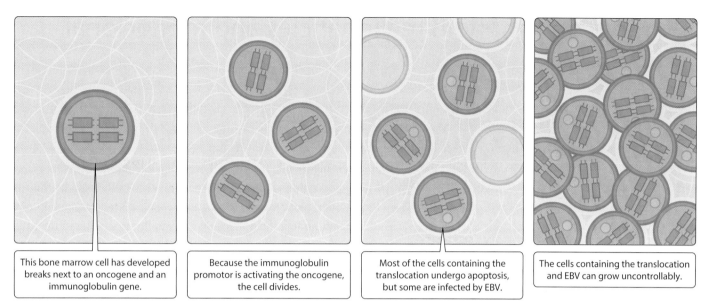

| | | | |
|---|---|---|---|
| This bone marrow cell has developed breaks next to an oncogene and an immunoglobulin gene. | Because the immunoglobulin promotor is activating the oncogene, the cell divides. | Most of the cells containing the translocation undergo apoptosis, but some are infected by EBV. | The cells containing the translocation and EBV can grow uncontrollably. |

**Fig. 3.37.2** Like most cancers, several events are required before lymphocytes can give rise to lymphoid malignancies. Here, there has been a chromosomal translocation and infection with Epstein–Barr virus.

Viruses can also contribute to lymphoid malignancies. Epstein–Barr virus is very common and causes glandular fever on initial infection. Like most herpesviruses, it has mechanisms for evading the immune system and surviving inside cells—in this case B cells. Epstein–Barr virus (EBV) produces proteins, encoded by viral oncogenes, that stimulate the uncontrolled growth of infected cells and protect against apoptosis. In most cases, two events are required for a lymphoid malignancy to develop. The first is a translocation; the second is often transformation by EBV (Fig. 3.37.2).

T cell malignancy is rare, but when it occurs, it is often caused by human T lymphotrophic virus 1 (HTLV1). This virus encodes Tax protein, which has similar effects to IL-2 (T cell growth factor). HTLV1 is rare in the developed world.

Most lymphoid malignancies are derived from cells of B cell lineage. This is partly because EBV is much more common than HTLV1, but also because in addition to recombination, B cells undergo somatic hypermutation, which carries a risk of translocation.

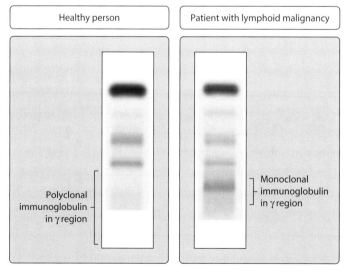

| Healthy person | Patient with lymphoid malignancy |
|---|---|

Polyclonal immunoglobulin in γ region

Monoclonal immunoglobulin in γ region

**Fig. 3.37.3** In a patient with a B cell malignancy there is a distinct band in the γ region on serum electrophoresis. This is because the malignant B cells are producing identical immunoglobulin molecules, which travel at the same speed in the gel.

# 38. More on lymphoid malignancies and monoclonal antibodies

**Questions**
- Describe the clinical features of acute lymphoblastic leukaemia, chronic lymphocytic leukaemia, lymphoma and myeloma.
- Explain how monoclonal antibodies are manufactured.

## CLINICAL FEATURES OF LYMPHOID MALIGNANCIES

Each of the different lymphoid malignances have different clinical characteristics. The exact characteristics depend on the cells from which they were originally derived (Fig. 3.38.1). The most serious lymphoid malignancy is **acute lymphoblastic leukaemia**, derived from very immature lymphocytes, most often of B cell lineage. The leukaemic cells (lymphoblasts) are rapidly dividing and are present in high numbers in the blood and bone marrow. Normal bone marrow function is impaired and there is a severe reduction in red cells, platelets and neutrophils: bone marrow failure. Cytotoxic chemotherapy is used to kill the leukaemic cells but is often unable to do this completely. If a few cells survive, they will continue to proliferate and the leukaemia then relapses. One way of effectively treating the leukaemia is to give such high doses of cytotoxic chemotherapy that all bone marrow cells are killed. A

stem cell transplant is then required if the patient is to survive (Chapter 42).

More mature B cells can give rise to less-aggressive malignancies. In **chronic lymphocytic leukaemia**, there is a large population of monoclonal mature cells in the blood. In many cases, chronic lymphocytic leukaemia does not cause symptoms and no treatment is required. **Lymphoma** is a solid tumour in which the malignant B cells are present mainly in lymph nodes. Early symptoms include swollen lymph nodes (lymphadenopathy). There are various types of lymphoma with varying severity. Some lymphomas are caused by Epstein–Barr virus and these are particularly common in patients with defective immune systems.

**Myeloma** is a malignancy of plasma cells and forms lesions in bone marrow. Myeloma cells secrete paraproteins, which are identified by electrophoresis (Fig. 3.37.3). The specific symptoms are of bone destruction; in addition, the paraprotein can cause kidney damage.

## MANUFACTURED MONOCLONAL ANTIBODIES

The perfect drug would be targeted against a specific cell type and have no effects on other cells. The potential to develop 'magic bullets' first arose in 1975 when **monoclonal antibodies**

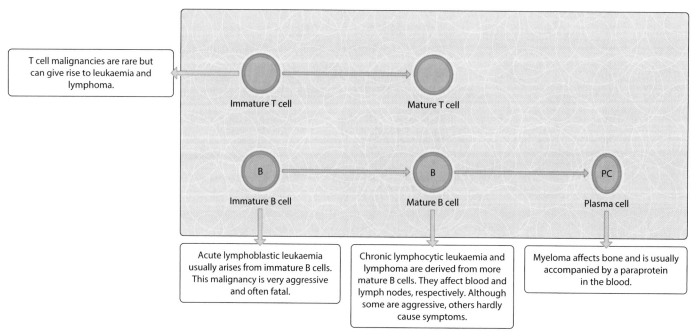

**Fig. 3.38.1** Each type of lymphoid malignancy develops from a different type of lymphocyte.

were developed in mice (Fig. 3.38.2). These are made by inoculating a mouse with the antigen of interest. For example, a malignant cell taken from a tumour could be used as antigen. Once antibodies are being produced, the B cells are immortalized by fusing them with rapidly dividing mouse myeloma cells. A single cell producing the highest affinity antibody is then selected and will rapidly produce many progeny cells. These cells will produce large quantities of monoclonal antibody that contains one identical immunoglobulin molecule.

Mouse monoclonal antibodies are not ideal for use as a treatment because they will eventually induce anti-mouse antibodies, and these can result in circulating immune-complex (type 3) hypersensitivity. To overcome this, the mouse myeloma cells can be genetically manipulated so that the Fc fragment (Chapter 16) only contains human amino acid sequences.

Monoclonal antibodies that block TNF are very effective at treating rheumatoid arthritis (Chapter 36). The most widely used TNF-blocking drug, **infliximab**, is an example of a **humanized monoclonal antibody**. In this case, the monoclonal antibody binds to TNF and prevents it from interacting with TNF receptors; this is a type of neutralization. You will read of some other examples of therapeutic monoclonal antibodies in the next few chapters.

## LYMPHOMA

A bacterial infection can give rise to lymphadenopathy (see Chapter 22). If lymphadenopathy persists when there is no obvious infection, lymphoma needs to be considered. A biopsy is often used to confirm this condition.

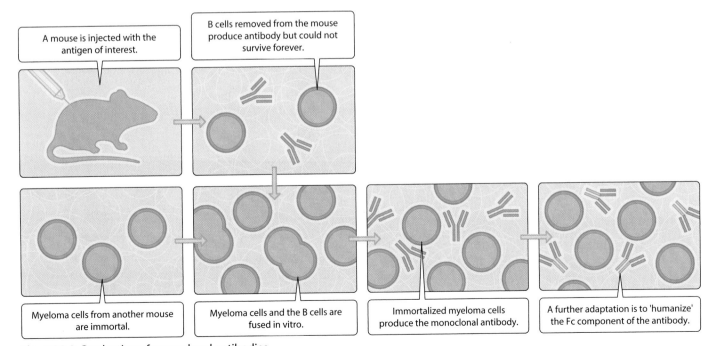

A mouse is injected with the antigen of interest.

B cells removed from the mouse produce antibody but could not survive forever.

Myeloma cells from another mouse are immortal.

Myeloma cells and the B cells are fused in vitro.

Immortalized myeloma cells produce the monoclonal antibody.

A further adaptation is to 'humanize' the Fc component of the antibody.

**Fig. 3.38.2** Production of monoclonal antibodies.

# 39. Immunity to tumours

## Questions

- Which tumours are most common in patients with defective immune systems? What is special about these tumours?
- How can mutations and translocations in cancer cells give rise to proteins that stimulate the immune system and help cancer cells to evade the immune system?
- Compare immunoglobulin and T cell immunotherapy for tumours.

## ■ IMMUNE RESPONSES TO TUMOURS

As we discussed in The Big Picture, the immune system evolved to deal with infections. Much research has been carried out to see if the immune system also surveys for and attacks tumours. Some tumours are 100 times commoner in patients with defective immune systems. These tumours include lymphoma, Kaposi sarcoma and carcinoma of the cervix. If the immunodeficiency can be improved, the tumours can regress. You will read more about this in subsequent sections. This has led some researchers to think that the immune system does combat tumours.

However, most of the tumours immunodeficient patients develop are driven by viruses (Epstein–Barr virus, human herpesvirus 8 and papilloma virus, respectively, for lymphoma,

Kaposi sarcoma and cervical carcinoma). So it is not clear if the immune system is responding to the tumour itself or to these oncogenic viruses. The vast majority of tumours are not caused by viruses but are the result of genetic damage caused by chemicals or radiation. There is less evidence that the immune system responds to this kind of tumour.

Most cancers do not produce novel proteins that would be recognized by the host immune system (Fig. 3.39.1). They occasionally produce normal host proteins at very high level, but in any case, the immune system becomes tolerant to these. In the rare instances where a novel protein is produced by a tumour cell (for example through a mutation or translocation), an immune response could then develop. There is some evidence that novel proteins produced by tumour cells do sometimes stimulate an immune response. However, if a tumour cell develops a second mutation that reduces HLA expression, it will escape the immune response. The cancer cell with a low level of HLA will have an advantage over other cells, which can be killed normally, and become the dominant cell type. This type of immune evasion may be important, because up to 50% of tumour cells express low levels of HLA. Finally, unlike infections, tumours do not activate a danger signal. Regardless of whether an abnormal protein is being produced and whether it can be presented, the immune system will not respond if there is no danger signal.

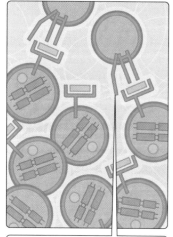

This patient has an EBV-driven lymphoma. Cytotoxic T cells recognize the EBV antigens.

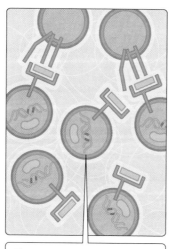

This cancer is caused by a mutation. The novel peptide that is produced is recognized by cytotoxic T cells.

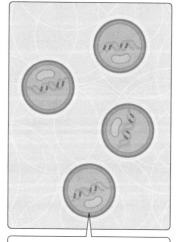

This cancer is caused by a mutation giving rise to a novel protein. However, a second mutation is preventing HLA being expressed. There is no immune response.

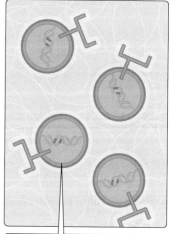

Although this cancer is caused by a mutation in a gene promoter, a new protein is not produced and there is no immune response.

**Fig. 3.39.1** A few tumour peptides encoded by viral genes or mutations are recognized by the immune system. Mostly, either the peptide is not recognized as foreign or it cannot be presented normally.

## ■ IMMUNOTHERAPY OF TUMOURS

If the immune system does not normally respond to tumours, is there any way the immune system can be used in **tumour immunotherapy**? The innate immune system can be stimulated by drugs that bind on to Toll-like receptors (see Chapter 2). For example, CpG binds Toll-like receptors and stimulates the production of a danger signal. CpG has been effective in the treatment of some tumours. Two main approaches have been used in the adaptive immune system to attack tumours. The first is passive immunotherapy, when a pre-existing immune entity is given to the patient. The second is when an immune entity is conjugated to an anti-tumour molecule.

Monoclonal antibodies are effective against some tumours. For example, an anti-B cell antibody called rituximab is effective in about 50% of cases of some lymphomas. The antibodies opsonize the tumour cells and stimulate phagocytosis (Fig. 3.39.1). Monoclonal antibodies can also be conjugated to a potent toxin, such as ricin or a radioactive isotope such as yttrium. Rituximab conjugated to yttrium has a better response rate, of about 80%.

In general, T cell responses to tumours cannot easily be boosted. In the laboratory, cellular immunity to tumours can be increased with cytokines. However, cytokines that activate T cells, such as IL-2, are too toxic to administer directly to patients. It is also possible to remove T cells from the body and activate them in the laboratory. These can be a random selection of T cells from the blood or T cells that have migrated specifically into the tumour. After activation, the cells are infused back into the patient; this approach has been successful in some cases. There is some evidence that **activated killer cells** are effective against tumours, but each treatment needs to be tailor-made for individual patients.

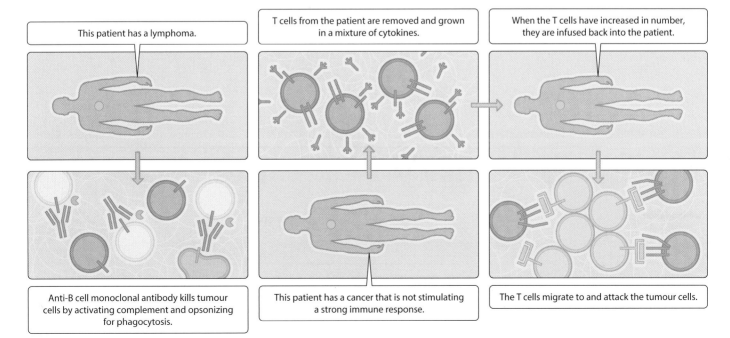

This patient has a lymphoma.

T cells from the patient are removed and grown in a mixture of cytokines.

When the T cells have increased in number, they are infused back into the patient.

Anti-B cell monoclonal antibody kills tumour cells by activating complement and opsonizing for phagocytosis.

This patient has a cancer that is not stimulating a strong immune response.

The T cells migrate to and attack the tumour cells.

**Fig. 3.39.2** Tumour therapy.

# 40. Transplantation: general concepts

## Questions
- Explain the terms syngeneic, allogeneic, xenogeneic, haploidentical and minor mismatch.
- Describe three ways by which the adaptive immune system recognizes allogeneic HLA antigens.

## DEFINITIONS

The immune system will usually reject tissue that has been transplanted at random from one individual to another because **alloreactive** T cells or antibodies recognize **alloantigens** in the transplanted tissue.

The risk of rejection depends on the difference between the donor and recipient: **autologous** and **syngeneic** transplant refer to transplants from one part of the body to another or between identical twins, respectively. These transplants do not carry a risk of rejection. **Allogeneic** transplant takes place between genetically non-identical members of the same species; there is always a risk of rejection (Fig. 3.40.1). **Xenogeneic** transplant takes place between different species and carries the highest risk of rejection.

## GENETICS

The key antigens that trigger alloreactions are the HLA antigens. You will remember from Chapter 13 that the other name for the HLA genes is the major histocompatibility complex (meaning compatibility between tissues). The HLA or MHC genes (A, B, C, DQ, DR and DP) are inherited in a block called a **haplotype**.

Some tissues, for example a single kidney or stem cells, can be transplanted from living donors. Very few people have identical twins who could act as donors, so the chances are they will have to rely on allogeneic transplantation. There is a 1:4 chance that a sibling will be HLA identical. Both parents and half the siblings will share half their HLA genes with the recipient: this is referred to as being **haploidentical**. Because the other halves of the HLA genes are different, haploidentical tissue will trigger an allogeneic response. For these reasons, large pools of unrelated donors are more likely to supply organs which are HLA identical or only have a minor mismatch.

## ALLOGENEIC REACTIONS

The polymorphisms in the HLA genes affect the amino acid sequence of the HLA peptides, and thus the surface structure of

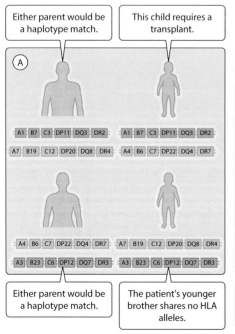

Either parent would be a haplotype match.

This child requires a transplant.

| A1 | B7 | C3 | DP11 | DQ3 | DR2 |   | A1 | B7 | C3 | DP11 | DQ3 | DR2 |
| A7 | B19 | C12 | DP20 | DQ8 | DR4 |   | A4 | B6 | C7 | DP22 | DQ4 | DR7 |

| A4 | B6 | C7 | DP22 | DQ4 | DR7 |   | A7 | B19 | C12 | DP20 | DQ8 | DR4 |
| A3 | B23 | C6 | DP12 | DQ7 | DR3 |   | A3 | B23 | C6 | DP12 | DQ7 | DR3 |

Either parent would be a haplotype match.

The patient's younger brother shares no HLA alleles.

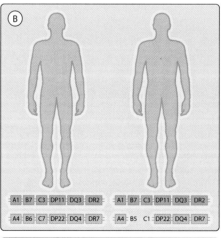

| A1 | B7 | C3 | DP11 | DQ3 | DR2 |   | A1 | B7 | C3 | DP11 | DQ3 | DR2 |
| A4 | B6 | C7 | DP22 | DQ4 | DR7 |   | A4 | B5 | C1 | DP22 | DQ4 | DR7 |

These donors have been identified from a panel. One donor happens to be HLA identical. The other has a minor mismatch only.

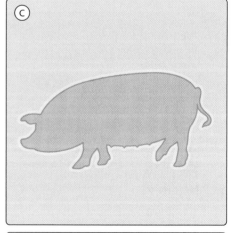

A pig would have very different proteins and sugars compared to the patient.

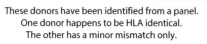

**Fig. 3.40.1** The child requiring a transplant is not going to get a good HLA match from family members (**A**). Unrelated donors could provide a better matched organ (**B**). A xenotransplant from a different species (**C**) would be the risky procedure.

the HLA protein. These differences in HLA surfaces are enough for them to act as macromolecular antigens recognized by antibody (Fig. 3.40.2). The production of anti-HLA antibodies requires priming, which can occur during pregnancy or after blood transfusion. Pregnant women are exposed to HLA antigens inherited by the fetus from its father. Unlike anti-D antibodies in haemolytic disease of the newborn, anti-HLA antibodies very rarely cause problems.

T cells that react to self-HLA antigen (without peptide antigen) are destroyed by negative selection in the thymus. However, it is possible for T cells to recognize non-self-HLA in two ways:

- the non-self-HLA molecule may through chance resemble self-HLA plus antigenic peptide
- the allogeneic HLA peptides themselves may undergo antigen processing and may be presented in the groove of a self-HLA molecule, just like any other foreign protein.

These T cell responses also require priming, although this very rarely takes place before transplantation.

It is also possible for a reaction to take place even after an HLA identical organ has been transplanted. This is because there are other allele systems, called the **minor histocompatibility antigens**.

## TRANSPLANTED ORGANS

Most kidneys are transplanted from brain-dead (cadaveric) donors. The chances of a random cadaveric donor being HLA identical are very small. This means that most people needing transplants will have to go on a waiting list before they receive their organ. Very often, the wait for an HLA-identical organ is so long that a patient will be offered an organ from a donor that differs at just one or two HLA loci: a **partial mismatch**. This still has a better chance of success than a haploidentical organ transplanted from a living sibling or a parent.

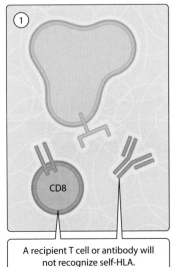

A recipient T cell or antibody will not recognize self-HLA.

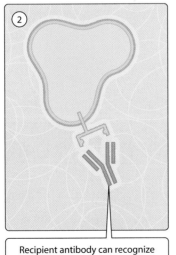

Recipient antibody can recognize donor HLA because its surface has a different structure.

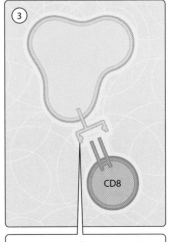

Recipient T cells may recognize the different amino acid sequence of 'empty' donor HLA.

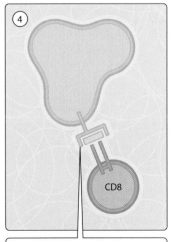

Donor HLA may be processed by recipient cells and presented as recipient HLA.

**Fig. 3.40.2** Alloantigen can be recognized in a variety of ways, each of which requires priming.

# 41. Transplantation rejection

### Questions
■ Describe three types of kidney transplant rejection.
■ What tests are done before transplant takes place to reduced the risk of rejection?

## ■ KIDNEY TRANSPLANTATION

The most commonly transplanted organs are the kidneys and the majority come from cadaveric donors. Three types of rejection can take place following kidney transplant: hyperacute, acute and chronic (Fig. 3.41.1).

### Hyperacute rejection

Hyperacute rejection takes place within minutes of the transplant if the recipient has high titres of anti-HLA or anti-ABO antibodies. This can only happen if the transplant recipient has been primed by previous pregnancy, blood transfusion or transplant. Antibody binding to endothelial cells triggers a type 2 hypersensitivity reaction. There is rapid blood vessel damage and the graft is destroyed by thrombosis.

### Acute rejection

Acute reaction is caused by T cells responding to HLA antigens and can happen within days or weeks of transplantation. The risk of acute rejection is related to the degree of mismatching, especially at HLA-DR loci. Even a single HLA allele mismatch can trigger acute rejection.

Acute rejection is a type 4 cell-mediated, delayed hypersensitivity reaction. Acute rejection takes several days to develop because of the time taken for donor dendritic cells to stimulate an allogeneic response and for responding T cells to proliferate and migrate into the donor kidney. The innate system is also activated during acute rejection, for example by damage done to the kidney after it is removed from the donor and before it is inserted into the recipient.

### Chronic rejection

Chronic rejection takes place months or years after transplant. Part of the problem is repeated bouts of low-level acute rejection. Autoimmune disease is a common cause of kidney disease (see Chapters 30, 33 and 34) and it may recur after transplant.

## ■ KIDNEY TRANSPLANT SCHEMES

Kidney transplant schemes operate across countries to maximize the chance of a recipient getting as closely matched a kidney as possible. When a patient first goes on the transplant waiting list, genetic tests are done to determine their HLA type: this referred to as **HLA typing**. The patient then goes on a

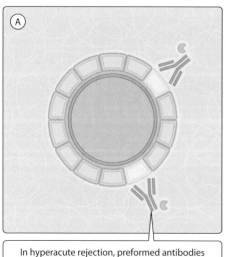

In hyperacute rejection, preformed antibodies bind to donor kidney cells and activate complement. Rejection occurs in minutes.

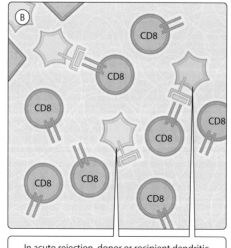

In acute rejection, donor or recipient dendritic cells with donor antigen migrate to a lymph node and prime T cells. T cells proliferate in response. Rejection takes several days to develop.

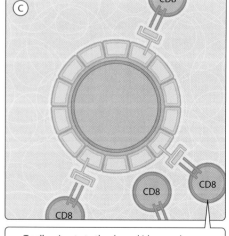

T cells migrate to the donor kidney and cause local damage.

**Fig. 3.41.1** Mechanisms causing hyperacute and acute rejection. In hyperacute rejection, pre-formed antibodies damage transplanted cells within minutes (**A**). In acute rejection, dendritic cells have to migrate to a local lymph node (**B**) and then T cells must migrate to the transplanted organ (**C**). This explains the delay in this type of rejection.

waiting list for as long as it takes for a kidney to become available. Dialysis keeps patients alive as they wait for a kidney transplant. If a suitable match becomes available, it is sent to the recipient's centre, along with a sample of donor white cells. The donor white cells and recipient plasma are tested to exclude any pre-existing anti-HLA antibodies, which could otherwise cause a hyperacute rejection (Fig. 3.41.2). If there are no antibodies, the kidney is transplanted as soon as possible.

## Rejection prophylaxis and treatment

Effective cross-matching should eliminate the risk of hyperacute rejection. Despite the efforts of the transplant schemes, most kidney transplants still take place with a minor HLA mismatch. Even when HLA is perfectly matched, minor histocompatibility antigens cause acute graft rejection in up to a third of transplants. For these reasons, patients are given immuno-suppressive drugs (described in Chapter 43) in an attempt to prevent acute graft rejection. Despite all these measures, acute rejection does take place following about 10% of transplants. If this happens, the dose of the immunosuppressive drugs is increased, or even more potent drugs are introduced.

### HEART TRANSPLANTS

When a patient desperately requires a heart transplant, there is often no alternative but to go ahead and give the transplant regardless of whether the donated organ is a perfect match. Because heart transplants are done without good HLA matching, patients need to be treated with very strong immunosuppressive drugs from the time of transplantation.

This patient has kidney failure. After being HLA typed he is placed on the transplant waiting list.

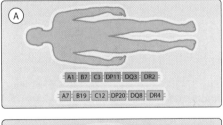

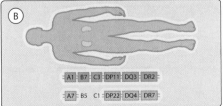

This person has had a traffic accident and is brain dead. His family have asked if he can be a kidney donor and he is HLA typed.

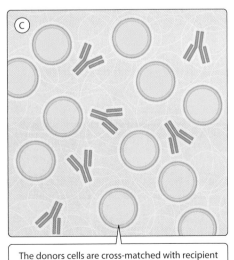

The donors cells are cross-matched with recipient serum to check there are no antibodies.

Because there is a two-allele HLA mismatch, immunosuppressive drugs are used to prevent rejection.

**Fig. 3.41.2** Several steps are taken to reduce the risk of kidney transplant rejection for the patient shown in (**A**). Only donors with identical HLA or a slight mismatch (**B**) are used. The cross-match is used to make sure the recipient has no pre-existing antibodies (**C**). Immunosuppressive drugs are used after the transplant (**D**).

# 42. Stem cell transplant

## Questions
- What are stem cells?
- Describe two types of stem cell transplant
- What is graft-versus-host disease?
- What are stem cell registries?

## ◼ HAEMATOPOIETIC STEM CELLS

Stem cells have two special characteristics: they are self-renewing and pluripotent. Self-renewing cells are able to divide constantly and replace themselves. Pluripotent cells can give rise to many different types of specialized cell.

From early in life, **haematopoietic stem cells** are found in bone marrow and, in lower numbers, in blood. These cells give rise to the red cells, lymphocytes, phagocytes, degranulating cells and platelets. Which cells are produced by haematopoietic stem cells depends on which cytokines are being secreted (Fig. 3.42.1); for example, during a bacterial infection, granulocyte colony-stimulating factor (G-CSF) is secreted and stimulates production of neutrophils (Chapter 5). During worm infection, IL-3 and IL-5 favour the production of eosinophils. There is some evidence that under certain circumstances, haematopoietic stem cells can produce other types of cell, for example skin or liver cells.

Stem cell transplant is used to treat two types of disease. The first is malignancies that require very potent cytotoxic chemotherapy in order to eliminate the malignant cells. The chemotherapy may irreversibly damage the patient's bone marrow, which can then be rescued with stem cell transplantation. Stem cell transplant is also used in genetic diseases affecting any of the types of cell mentioned above, for example in severe combined immunodeficiency (SCID; Chapter 47).

### Stem cell transplant

Stem cells can be obtained from donor bone marrow or blood. To get adequate numbers of cells from blood, the donor has to be given G-CSF before the stem cells can be harvested. Stem cells can also be obtained from cord blood, which would otherwise be discarded after the umbilicus has been cut. Before the transplant can take place, cytotoxic drugs are given to destroy the recipient's bone marrow and create space for the incoming stem cells.

Stem cells can be rejected by the recipient immune system, as for solid organ transplantation described in the previous section. Before transplant can take place, a donor with a close as possible HLA type must be found and the cross-match must be negative. Depending on the degree of HLA or 'minor' antigen mismatch, patients undergoing stem cell transplant are given immunosuppressive drugs to prevent rejection (Fig. 3.42.2).

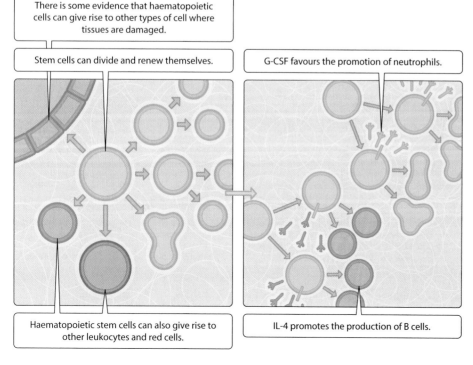

There is some evidence that haematopoietic cells can give rise to other types of cell where tissues are damaged.

Stem cells can divide and renew themselves.

G-CSF favours the promotion of neutrophils.

Haematopoietic stem cells can also give rise to other leukocytes and red cells.

IL-4 promotes the production of B cells.

**Fig. 3.42.1** Stem cells provide a flexible and renewable source of cells. The type of cell produced depends on which cytokines are being secreted.

An important difference between solid organ and stem cell transplant is that donor T cells can mount an allogeneic response against the host, causing **graft-versus-host disease**. The donor T cells attack recipient tissues causing damage, which is often fatal. The chances of graft-versus-host disease are reduced by careful HLA matching and by the use of immunosuppressive drugs.

HLA-identical family members are not often available for stem cell transplant (see Fig. 3.40.1). **Stem cell registries** are lists of potential donors who have been HLA typed (Fig. 3.42.3). The donors have all agreed to donate bone marrow if a patient requires bone marrow of their HLA type.

## INFECTION AFTER STEM CELL TRANSPLANT

Even when there is a good HLA match between donor and recipient, up to 20% of recipients may die. Infection is the most serious problem after stem cell transplant, partly because of the deliberate destruction of bone marrow before transplant and partly because of the immunosuppressive drugs given afterwards. For the first few weeks, there are very few neutrophils being produced by the bone marrow. T and B cells take even longer to recover from stem cell transplant. During this phase, patients are given antibiotics to reduce the risk of infection.

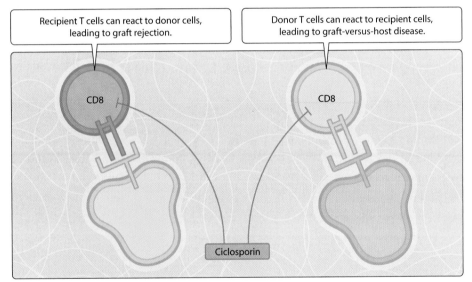

Recipient T cells can react to donor cells, leading to graft rejection.

Donor T cells can react to recipient cells, leading to graft-versus-host disease.

CD8

CD8

Ciclosporin

**Fig. 3.42.2** Immunosuppressive drugs are used to prevent both graft rejection and graft-versus-host disease after stem cell transplant.

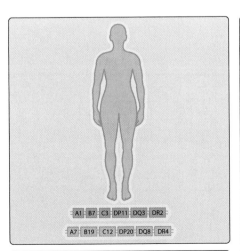

| A1 | B7 | C3 | DP11 | DQ3 | DR2 |
| A7 | B19 | C12 | DP20 | DQ8 | DR4 |

This patient has leukaemia and requires a stem cell transplant. She has been HLA typed.

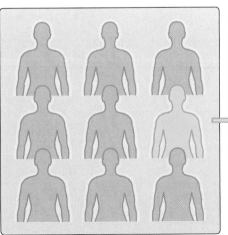

An HLA identical donor is found from a stem cell registry.

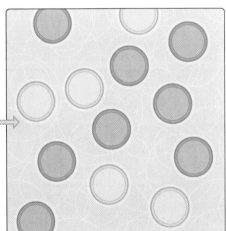

For stem cell transplant, the cross-match procedure excludes reactions between donor and recipient T cells.

**Fig. 3.42.3** Registries are increasingly being used to identify stem cell donors.

# 43. Immunosuppressive drugs and xenotransplantation

## Questions
- When are immunosuppressive drugs used?
- Describe four classes of anti-T cell drug?
- Which two immunological problems may transgenic pigs overcome?

## ■ IMMUNOSUPPRESSIVE DRUGS

Immunosuppressive drugs are used to treat hypersensitivity to a range of antigens, including autoimmunity (self-antigen), allergy (harmless environmental antigen) and transplantation reactions (alloantigen). The ideal immunosuppressive drug would only inhibit responses to the specific antigens involved, in other words achieve a state of tolerance. In practice, specific tolerance is almost impossible to achieve and most drugs also suppress immune responses to pathogens and therefore increase the risk of infection.

Corticosteroids are used widely as immunosuppressive drugs, although they have very many side effects because they affect very many different types of cell (Chapter 36). More recently developed drugs have specific effects on T cells and so can be more potent, with fewer side effects. These drugs either prevent T cells from responding to antigen in the first place or prevent T cell proliferation after antigen stimulation. Four classes of

drug that act against T cells are used in the prevention and treatment of hypersensitivity reactions such as acute graft rejection (Fig. 3.43.1).

- **Ciclosporin** and **tacrolimus** interact with immunophilins and prevent signalling molecules from functioning after the T cell receptor has been triggered (Chapter 11). T cells that cannot signal through the T cell receptor are unable to respond to antigen.
- Once T cell signalling has taken place, T cells secrete IL-2, which acts as a growth factor for T cells. **Basiliximab** is a monoclonal antibody against the IL-2 receptor. If IL-2 is unable to bind to its receptor, T cells are unable to proliferate.
- **Rapamycin** inhibits signals after IL-2 has bound to its receptor. It binds to a protein kinase specifically activated by IL-2 binding to its receptor.
- **Mycophenolate** and **azathioprine** inhibit proliferation of many types of cell, but particularly T cells.

### INFECTIONS WITH IMMUNOSUPPRESSIVE DRUGS

All immunosuppressive drugs increase the risk of infection. The more potent the drug, the higher the risk of infection. These drugs also increase the risk of malignancies caused by infection, especially lymphoma driven by Epstein–Barr virus.

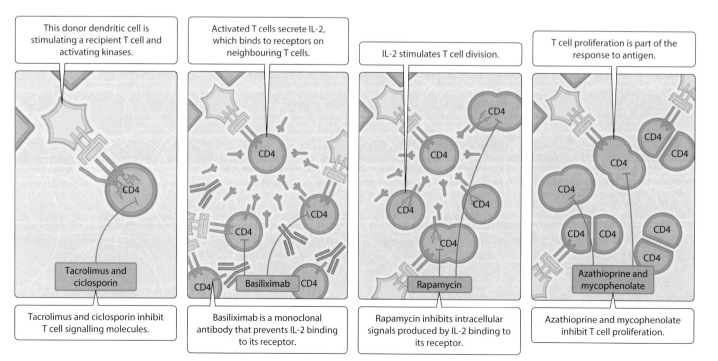

This donor dendritic cell is stimulating a recipient T cell and activating kinases.

Tacrolimus and ciclosporin

Tacrolimus and ciclosporin inhibit T cell signalling molecules.

Activated T cells secrete IL-2, which binds to receptors on neighbouring T cells.

Basiliximab

Basiliximab is a monoclonal antibody that prevents IL-2 binding to its receptor.

IL-2 stimulates T cell division.

Rapamycin

Rapamycin inhibits intracellular signals produced by IL-2 binding to its receptor.

T cell proliferation is part of the response to antigen.

Azathioprine and mycophenolate

Azathioprine and mycophenolate inhibit T cell proliferation.

**Fig. 3.43.1** Modern immunosuppressive drugs specifically inhibit T cell signalling and proliferation.

# ■ XENOTRANSPLANTATION

There are too few human organs available to meet the needs of patients: waiting times for kidney transplants double every 10 years, while the number of transplants carried out remains static. The use of non-primate (for example pig) organs could surmount this difficulty, but several problems prevent **xenotransplants** being a practical alternative (Fig. 3.43.2).

- Primates and non-primates use very different sugars on the surfaces of cells. Non-primates use similar sugars to gut bacteria. Humans produce natural antibodies to non-primate sugars following exposure to gut bacteria (mentioned in Chapter 20). Antibodies against non-primate sugars bind onto xenotransplanted organs, activate complement and trigger hyperacute rejection.

- Cell surfaces act as a platform for the spontaneous breakdown of complement component C3. This is the basis of the alternative pathway of complement activation (Chapter 3). Human cells express complement inhibitor to prevent on-going complement activation. Pig cells promote the alternative pathway because pig inhibitors will not inhibit human complement; widespread complement activation leads to destruction of the transplanted tissue.

Genetic techniques are being used to create pigs that express only primate-type sugars and also human-type complement inhibitors. Although there may be other problems to be overcome, these **transgenic pigs** may help to relieve the human organ shortage.

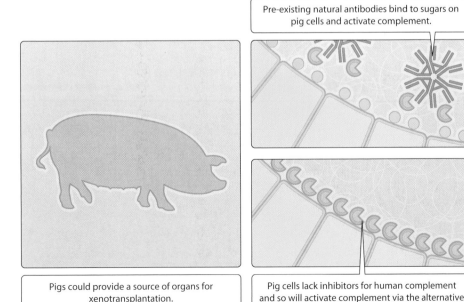

Pre-existing natural antibodies bind to sugars on pig cells and activate complement.

**Fig. 3.43.2** Obstacles to xenotransplantation.

Pigs could provide a source of organs for xenotransplantation.

Pig cells lack inhibitors for human complement and so will activate complement via the alternative pathway, even in the absence of antibodies.

# 44. Vaccines

## Questions
- How do antibodies induced by vaccines prevent infectious disease?
- How can the immunogenicity of vaccines be improved?
- How does boosting improve vaccine responses?

## ■ PRINCIPLES OF VACCINATION

Vaccines have eradicated some infections, preventing millions of deaths from, for example, smallpox. For other important infections, there are still no effective vaccines.

Effective vaccines reduce the risk of an infectious disease taking place. Vaccines induce a primary adaptive immune response in the host, thereby establishing immunological memory. When the host is re-exposed, a secondary response develops. The secondary response is rapid and includes high levels of high-affinity antibody. This **active immunity** is very different from **passive immunity**, where immunity is transferred from one person to another (Chapter 15).

Antibodies induced by vaccines can prevent infection taking place in the first place (Fig. 3.44.1). For example, antibodies against the influenza haemagglutinin molecule can prevent this virus from binding onto its target cells (Chapter 15). Other vaccines induce antibodies that opsonize pathogens or promote antibody-dependent cellular cytotoxicity (Chapter 17). Other vaccines induce antibodies that may not prevent an infection from taking place but prevent the infection from causing harm.

For example, antibodies against tetanus toxin prevent tetanus developing after *Clostridium tetani* infection (Chapter 15).

The effectiveness of antibody at preventing many infections explains why most current vaccines aim to produce memory B and Th2 cells, which together produce high-titre antibody on exposure to the pathogen or its toxin. Very few existing vaccines aim to produce Th1 responses. A notable example is the vaccinia vaccine against smallpox.

Vaccines elicit adaptive immune responses in just the same ways as pathogens. On initial exposure (priming), antigen is conveyed to the lymph node by dendritic cells. The dendritic cells need to be stimulated by an innate immune system danger signal. Some vaccines do this by including a live organism that reproduces in vivo and will trigger innate responses by producing double-stranded RNA or bacterial polysaccharides. These vaccines tend to elicit the best kind of response. Other vaccines contain whole dead organisms. Polysaccharides and lipids from the dead organism trigger weaker danger signals (Fig. 3.44.2).

Vaccines containing only peptide components of pathogens (subunit vaccines) do not produce a danger signal and will not induce a good immune response. Subunit vaccines can be combined with dead organisms to improve the response.

Another strategy is to add an adjuvant. An **adjuvant** is a chemical that directly causes low-grade inflammation, thus activating the innate immune system and providing a danger signal. Aluminium salts (alum) are the only licenced adjuvant currently in use in the UK. CpG is also being tested as an adjuvant.

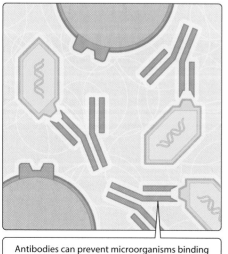

Antibodies can prevent microorganisms binding to receptors on cells, e.g. influenza virus.

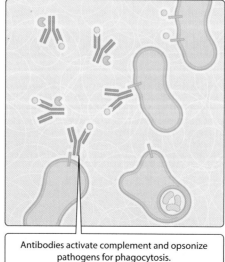

Antibodies activate complement and opsonize pathogens for phagocytosis.

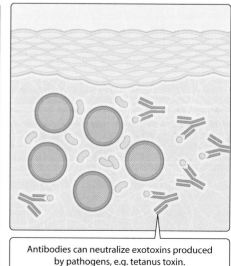

Antibodies can neutralize exotoxins produced by pathogens, e.g. tetanus toxin.

**Fig. 3.44.1** Antibodies elicited by vaccines prevent infectious disease in a number of ways.

The initial vaccination usually induces only weak responses and poor immunological memory. Vaccine **boosters** improve antibody titres by somatic hypermutation and sustain the duration of immunological memory (Chapter 19). Most vaccines require several boosters when first given. Boosters are sometimes given again after several years. For example, tetanus vaccine is given three times during infancy and boosted at school entry and school leaving. People who have injuries are also given a booster, if they have not had one for 10 years (Table 44.1).

### UK VACCINE STRATEGY

Vaccine strategies must take into account the immunogenicity of different vaccines. For example, the purified proteins in the tetanus and diphtheria vaccines are not good at eliciting a danger signal from the innate immune system. Pertussis (whooping cough) vaccine contains a whole dead organism, which stimulates the innate immune system. When this is combined with the diphtheria and tetanus proteins, responses to these are improved.

**Table 44.1** A VACCINATION PROGRAMME SHOWING TIMES FOR FIRST VACCINE DOSE

| Age | Vaccine against | Type of vaccine |
| --- | --- | --- |
| 2 months | Diphtheria | Toxoid |
| | Tetanus | Toxoid |
| | Pertussis | Dead organism |
| | *Haemophilus* | Conjugated polysaccharide |
| | *Meningococcus* C | Conjugated polysaccharide |
| | Polio | Live attenuated |
| 1 year | Measles | Live attenuated |
| | Mumps | Live attenuated |
| | Rubella | Live attenuated |
| 10–14 years | Tuberculosis (BCG) | Live attenuated |
| Elderly and high-risk patients | Influenza | Dead organism |

Live vaccines, usually attenuated viruses, reproduce inside cells.

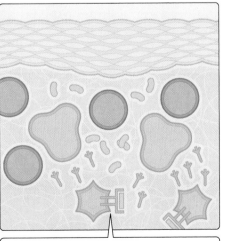

Live vaccines elicit innate immune system danger signals, such as interferon. These signals stimulate dendritic cells to migrate to lymph nodes and then help to stimulate T cells.

Dead vaccines elicit weak danger signals, for example when macrophages recognize sugars on the surface of dead bacteria.

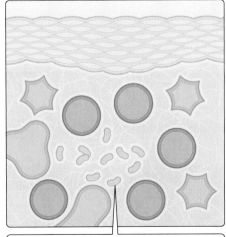

Vaccines made of peptide components of pathogens do not elicit danger signals unless an adjuvant is added.

**Fig. 3.44.2** Different types of vaccine have variable **immunogenicity**, partly dependent on whether or not they induce a danger signal.

# 45. Types of vaccine

## Questions
- What are the advantages and disadvantages of live attenuated, killed and subunit vaccine?
- How does HLA type affect the response to hepatitis B vaccine?
- How do conjugate vaccines promote antibodies against encapsulated bacteria?
- What are the risks of live polio vaccine?

## ■ LIVE ATTENUATED VACCINES

Attenuated vaccines contain pathogens that have been weakened so that they will not cause disease. Some vaccines use naturally occurring organisms. For example, vaccinia is a natural virus that causes the trivial cowpox infection. It shares antigens with the variola virus, which causes smallpox. After exposure to vaccinia, Th1 cells are produced and sterilizing immunity is achieved (Fig. 3.45.1a). The Th1 memory cells that recognize vaccinia peptides also recognize variola and protect against smallpox. Vaccinia was the first vaccine used and produces immunity against smallpox for many years. It was responsible for eradicating smallpox in the 1970s. Because of the threat of bioterrorism, it is now being used again.

Attenuated vaccines can also be artificially made using recombinant technology to develop completely new viruses, which may contain antigens from a range of different pathogens.

Live attenuated vaccines are good immunogens because they trigger danger signals during their life cycles. Because they live inside cells, peptides from live vaccines gain access to the antigen-presentation pathways and are presented on HLA class I molecules to stimulate cytotoxic T cells.

A disadvantage of live attenuated vaccines is that the organism may spontaneously revert back to the naturally occurring (**wild-type**) strain. For example, the genome for the attenuated polio vaccine differs from the wild-type vaccine by only ten base pairs. It is relatively easy for the attenuated vaccine to mutate back to the disease-causing wild-type virus. A second problem is that attenuated viruses are capable of growing and causing disease in immunodeficient patients (see Chapter 46).

## ■ DEAD VACCINES

Dead vaccines are safer than live attenuated vaccines because they cannot, of course, cause infection. However, because they do not reproduce or get inside cells, they are not such potent immunogens and they do not elicit cytotoxic T cell responses.

Influenza vaccine is a killed form that is given with an adjuvant to promote its immunogenicity. Because the influenza virus is constantly changing through drift and shift, vaccine manufacturers produce a new vaccine every year (Chapter 25).

## ■ SUBUNIT VACCINES

The three types of subunit vaccine do not, of course, replicate and rarely cause side effects. These vaccines always require adjuvants.

**Toxoid vaccines** are derived from bacterial exotoxins that have been chemically treated to make them safe, for

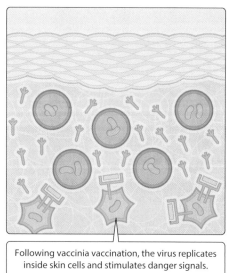

Following vaccinia vaccination, the virus replicates inside skin cells and stimulates danger signals.

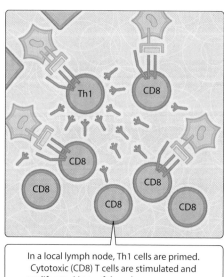

In a local lymph node, Th1 cells are primed. Cytotoxic (CD8) T cells are stimulated and proliferate. Many of these become memory cells and survive for years.

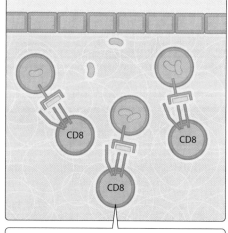

Small pox virus invades the respiratory epithelium. Memory T cells provide a rapid response and prevent the virus from establishing infection.

**Fig. 3.45.1** Vaccinia vaccine for small pox is one of the few vaccines that elicits a strong cytotoxic T cell response.

example tetanus toxoid vaccine. Although they do not prevent infection, they prevent the complications of infection from taking place.

**Recombinant subunit vaccines** contain synthetic peptides that act as extracellular antigens; they are phagocytosed, digested and then presented on HLA class II. Recombinant peptide vaccines contain only a limited number of possible antigen peptides. Through chance, some individuals may not have HLA class II molecules capable of binding these peptides and will not respond to the vaccine. This happens with recombinant hepatitis B vaccines. Although the vaccine has almost eradicated the virus in some countries, individuals with the 'wrong' HLA alleles cannot respond to it (Fig. 3.45.2).

*Pneumococcus, Haemophilus* and *Meningococcus* spp. produce polysaccharide capsules to evade antibodies. They can cause life-threatening infection in babies because T-independent B cells do not start producing anti-polysaccharide antibodies until later in childhood (Chapter 20 and 24). **Conjugate polysaccharide vaccines** combine protein antigens (for example tetanus toxoid) with the polysaccharide. Th2 cells responding to the protein component provide help for B cells, which can then respond well to the polysaccharide component (Fig. 3.45.3).

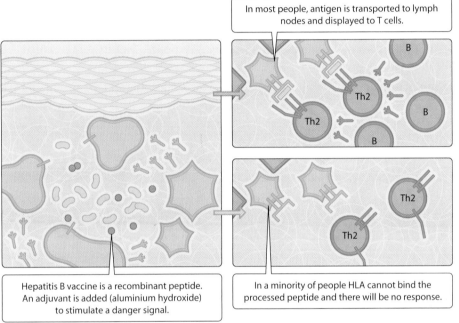

In most people, antigen is transported to lymph nodes and displayed to T cells.

Hepatitis B vaccine is a recombinant peptide. An adjuvant is added (aluminium hydroxide) to stimulate a danger signal.

In a minority of people HLA cannot bind the processed peptide and there will be no response.

**Fig. 3.45.2** Recombinant subunit vaccine requires HLA to present antigen.

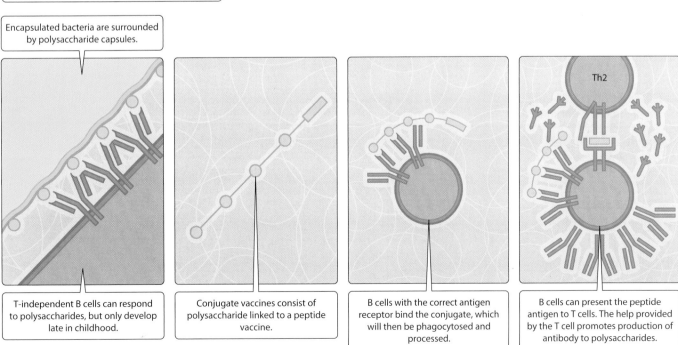

Encapsulated bacteria are surrounded by polysaccharide capsules.

T-independent B cells can respond to polysaccharides, but only develop late in childhood.

Conjugate vaccines consist of polysaccharide linked to a peptide vaccine.

B cells with the correct antigen receptor bind the conjugate, which will then be phagocytosed and processed.

B cells can present the peptide antigen to T cells. The help provided by the T cell promotes production of antibody to polysaccharides.

**Fig. 3.45.3** Conjugate vaccines use an antigenic component to enable a response to a non-antigenic molecule.

# 46. Immunodeficiency

**Questions**
- What are opportunist infections?
- How does the type of opportunist infection give clues to the severity and type of immunodeficiency?
- What is the difference between primary and secondary immunodeficiency?
- Name three causes of secondary immunodeficiency.

## ■ DEFINITION

Immunodeficiency is a state of impaired immunity, leading to an increased risk of infection and malignancy. The malignancies are generally driven by infection, for example Epstein–Barr virus-driven lymphoma. The infections that occur in immunodeficiency have specific characteristics.

- Immunodeficient patients have more infections than normal individuals; any infection can recur and there may be several infections at once.
- Infections also tend to be chronic, taking weeks, months or even years to be resolved.
- Immunodeficient patients develop infections with organisms that do not cause problems in normal individuals. These are called **opportunist infections**. Reactivation of *Mycobacterium tuberculosis* (Chapter 26) is an opportunist infection and

can occur in people with mild immunodeficiency. Patients with much more severe immunodeficiency may develop opportunist infection with normally harmless mycobacteria that live in the environment. The type of opportunist infection depends on the severity of the immunodeficiency.

As well as giving clues as to the *severity* of immunodeficiency (Fig. 3.46.1), the type of infection experienced by a patient also gives clues to the *type* of immunodeficiency. Defects in T cells, interferon or TNF cause infection with intracellular pathogens, such as viruses, protozoa and intracellular bacteria (e.g. mycobacteria). Other immune system components defend against extracellular infections. Defects in complement, phagocytes and antibody can all cause opportunist infections with extracellular pathogens, mainly bacteria. If a patient has recurrent bacterial infections, it is important to look for problems in complement, phagocytes and antibody (Fig. 3.46.2).

## ■ CAUSES OF IMMUNODEFICIENCY

Immunodeficiencies are classified as primary and secondary. **Primary immunodeficiencies** have a genetic basis and are caused by mutations in immune system genes. Primary immunodeficiencies are rare and tend to cause severe infections early in life. These problems are described in the next two chapters.

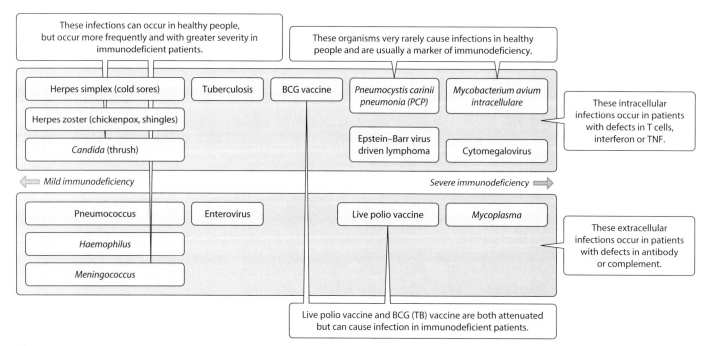

**Fig. 3.46.1** The species of infecting organism gives clues to the type and severity of immune deficiency.

**Secondary immunodeficiencies** are caused by problems that have been acquired during life. This includes some of the lymphoid malignancies mentioned in Chapter 37. Patients with myeloma or leukaemia very often have recurrent infections. This is because the resources and physical space available in the immune system are all being taken over by the malignant clone.

Drugs are another important cause of secondary immunodeficiency. Sometimes infections are an expected side effect. For example, immunosuppressive drugs (Chapter 43) commonly cause secondary immunodeficiency. These drugs often affect T cell function; consequently, intracellular opportunist infections are particularly common. Another class of drugs are the cytotoxics, which are used to treat cancer and to prepare for bone marrow transplantation. These drugs prevent cells from dividing. They very often affect the bone marrow and cause low levels of neutrophils (**neutropenia**). Neutropenic patients are very susceptible to opportunist bacterial infections.

The final type of secondary immunodeficiency is caused by HIV infection. This is so important that two later chapters are dedicated to it.

Note that secondary immunodeficiencies are much more common than primary immunodeficiencies. For example, neutropenia caused by drugs is relatively common, while defective neutrophil function caused by mutations (such as chronic granulomatous disease (Chapter 4) or leukocyte adhesion defect (Chapter 23)), are very rare.

### GENETIC PREDISPOSITION TO INFECTION

Apart from the very rare mutations causing primary immunodeficiencies, much commoner genetic polymorphisms also predispose to infection. For example, polymorphisms affecting mannose-binding lectin affect the risk of a wide range of infection (Chapter 2), while HLA polymorphisms tend to affect the risk of a few specific infections, such as HIV (Chapter 13). There may be many more genetic polymorphisms affecting the risk of infection, because during epidemics not everyone will become infected.

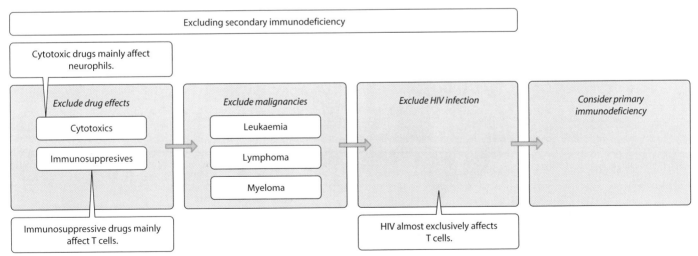

**Fig. 3.46.2** Investigation of patients with recurrent or severe infection.

# 47. Primary immunodeficiencies affecting antibody production

## Questions
- Describe two X-linked causes of antibody deficiency.
- Describe two polygenic causes of antibody deficiency.
- What is bronchiectasis?

## ■ CAUSES OF PRIMARY ANTIBODY DEFICIENCY

There are two main types of primary antibody deficiency: those caused by single mutations and those caused by the interaction of several genetic and environmental factors (Fig. 3.47.1).

- Antibody deficiency caused by single mutations can also be divided into two groups depending on where in the pathway of B cell production the defect occurs (Fig. 3.47.1). In **X-linked agammaglobulinaemia** (XLA), there is a mutation in the gene for a protein called BTK, on the X chromosome (Fig. 3.47.2). This protein is required for B cell maturation and affected boys usually have no B cells or immunoglobulin. Mutations affecting later stages of B cell maturation will result in selective loss of a particular immunoglobulin class. For example, mutations in the gene

for CD40 ligand, also on the X chromosome, prevent B cell class switching in the **hyper-IgM syndrome** (Chapter 19). Affected boys can produce IgM at high levels but they are unable to produce other immunoglobulin classes. Boys with hyper-IgM syndrome and XLA often remain well until they are about 6 months old. This is because IgG pumped across the placenta in the last few weeks of pregnancy will initially protect them from infection.

- Polygenic disorders are caused by the interaction of several genes, with a contribution from environmental factors. **Common variable immunodeficiency** (CVID) is a relatively common polygenic disorder mainly affecting antibody production. The mutations or polymorphisms causing CVID are not known. Patients with CVID have low levels of total IgG and variable levels of IgA and IgM.

  A related disorder is **specific antibody deficiency**. There is a failure of T-independent B cells to produce antibodies against polysaccharide-coated organisms (Chapter 23). The genetic causes for specific antibody deficiency and CVID are not known (Fig. 3.47.2). Environmental factors are also important and might include exposure to drugs or infections.

**Fig. 3.47.1** Stages of B cell development affected in antibody deficiencies.

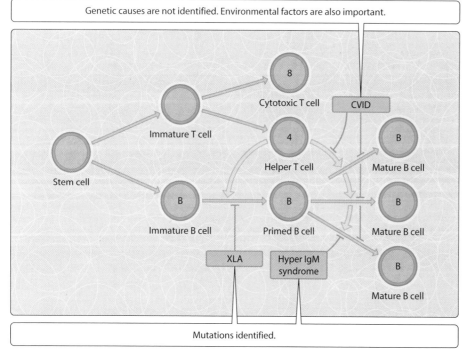

Genetic causes are not identified. Environmental factors are also important.

Stem cell

Immature T cell

8 — Cytotoxic T cell

CVID

4 — Helper T cell

B — Mature B cell

B — Immature B cell

B — Primed B cell

B — Mature B cell

B — Mature B cell

XLA

Hyper IgM syndrome

Mutations identified.

## CONSEQUENCES OF ANTIBODY DEFICIENCY

Patients with antibody deficiency are predisposed to infection with extracellular organisms, especially bacteria. Patients with antibody deficiency develop frequent, recurrent bacterial infections of the entire respiratory tract. Infections of the upper respiratory tract can lead to sinusitis or deafness. Infections of the lower respiratory tract initially lead to bouts of pneumonia. Each attack of infection causes scarring, particularly of the bronchial walls. Antibody deficiency is one cause of irreversible bronchial wall damage, referred to as **bronchiectasis**.

In addition, patients with antibody deficiency have problems dealing with viral infections. Remember that antibodies can prevent the initial phases of viral infection, although T cells are required to achieve sterilizing immunity. For example, if antibody-deficient patients are given live attenuated polio vaccine, they can develop chronic infection of the gut, presumably because they are unable to produce IgA. In this example, the attenuated polio virus is acting as an opportunist pathogen; it is not usually able to establish chronic infection or cause disease in normal individuals.

## TREATMENT

It is very important to prevent infections that cause irreversible damage. In some patients, this can be achieved by giving prophylactic (preventative) antibiotics. Many other patients require **immunoglobulin replacement**, which is given by intravenous or subcutaneous injection. Immunoglobulin is manufactured from donated plasma. Large volumes of plasma, from several thousand donors, are required to manufacture immunoglobulin. The immunoglobulin injections are given regularly for life. Because so many donors are required, immunoglobulin always carries a risk of transmitting blood-borne pathogens, such as hepatitis viruses.

### TRANSIENT ANTIBODY DEFICIENCY OF INFANCY

Not very much IgG is pumped across the placenta until the last few weeks of pregnancy. Normal infants do not start producing effective amounts of IgG until they are about 6 months old, when pathogens or vaccines have stimulated their B cells. If a child is born a few weeks prematurely, it will not have adequate maternal immunoglobulin and will have a high risk of bacterial infection for the first few months of life.

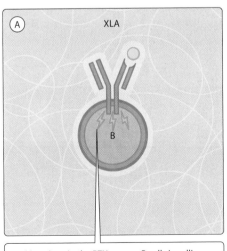

Mutations in the BTK gene, a B cell signalling molecule, prevents mature B cell formation.

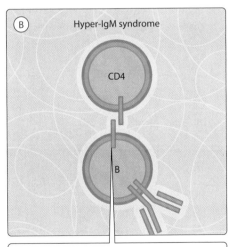

Mutations in the CD40 ligand gene prevents B cell communication with T cells during immunoglobulin class switching.

**Fig. 3.47.2** Causes of antibody deficiency diseases are not all known.

# 48. Primary immunodeficiencies causing T cell defects

## Questions
- What are the clinical features of Di George syndrome?
- Describe autosomal recessive and X-linked SCID.
- How can babies with SCID be protected from infection?
- Why is gene therapy more likely to work in SCID than in other genetic diseases?

## ■ CAUSES OF PRIMARY T CELL DEFECTS

There are two main types of T cell defect (Fig. 3.48.1). The first type cause absence of T cells. A good example is Di George syndrome (Chapter 12). The Di George syndrome is caused by developmental abnormalities of the third and fourth branchial arches, which give rise to the thymus, parathyroid glands and the aortic arch. These children have heart failure, problems with calcium metabolism, and primary immunodeficiency because they produce very low numbers of T cells. If T cells are missing, B cells will not function normally.

The second type of defect affects both T and B cells (Fig. 3.48.2). This group of disorders are called **severe combined immunodeficiency** (SCID). One cause of autosomal recessive SCID is defects in the recombinase genes required to generate both T and B cell receptors (Chapter 10). X-linked SCID is caused by a mutation that affects the receptors for IL-2 and IL-4. IL-2 is a growth factor for T and B cells (Chapter 11) and IL-4 stimulates B cell maturation (Chapter 19). If the receptors are deficient, T and B cell proliferation cannot take place and B cells cannot produce immunoglobulin.

## ■ CONSEQUENCES OF PRIMARY T CELL DEFECTS

Unlike children with antibody deficiency, patients with T cell defects develop infections soon after birth. This is because maternal T cells are not transferred across the placenta and there is no passive T cell immunity after birth. These children develop severe intracellular infections (viruses, protozoa, fungi and mycobacteria) soon after birth. Children with SCID are also susceptible to infection with organisms in attenuated vaccines.

## ■ TREATMENT OF SCID

Babies with SCID must be protected from infection by barrier nursing: 'the boy in the bubble' was an example of a child with SCID. This is not sustainable in the long term and, at the moment, stem cell transplant is the only curative procedure.

The majority of children with SCID do not have HLA identical siblings who could act as stem cell donors (though their production by in vitro fertilization is a controversial proposal). Public registries have been set up to provide stem cells for these children (Chapter 42). However, HLA is so polymorphic that even when there are several thousand volunteers on a register, a donor cannot always be found. In these cases, **gene therapy** may be an option (Fig. 3.48.3).

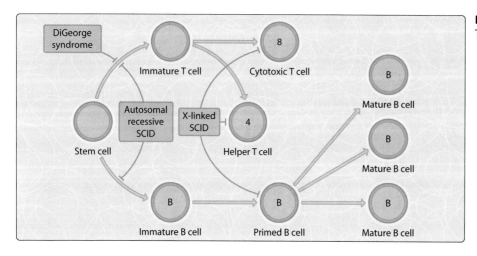

**Fig. 3.48.1** Effects of genetic diseases on T cell maturation.

## GENE THERAPY

Gene therapy has been tried in X-linked SCID. The corrected gene for the cytokine receptor is inserted into patient's stem cells. This process is called **transfection** and occurs at random in the genome (Fig. 3.48.3). Gene therapy is more likely to work in SCID than in other genetic diseases because:

- it is easy to get access to stem cells
- the transfected cells will proliferate rapidly and do not have to compete with other cells for space

- in other diseases, the immune system will recognize the protein encoded by the transfected gene as 'foreign' and mount an immune response; this will not happen in SCID.

Several boys with X-linked SCID have been successfully treated with gene therapy. Unfortunately, two of these boys subsequently developed T cell leukaemia. This is probably because the transfected gene and its promoter were inserted next to an oncogene in one clone of T cells.

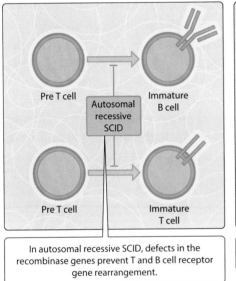

In autosomal recessive SCID, defects in the recombinase genes prevent T and B cell receptor gene rearrangement.

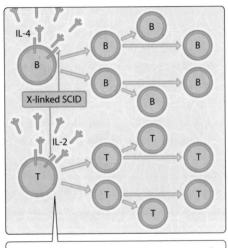

In X-linked SCID, there is a defect in the receptor for IL-4 and IL-2, the growth factors for B and T cells.

**Fig. 3.48.2** The molecular causes of autosomal recessive and X-linked SCID.

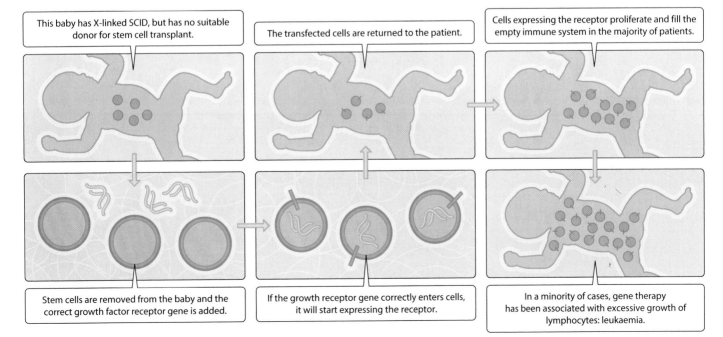

This baby has X-linked SCID, but has no suitable donor for stem cell transplant.

The transfected cells are returned to the patient.

Cells expressing the receptor proliferate and fill the empty immune system in the majority of patients.

Stem cells are removed from the baby and the correct growth factor receptor gene is added.

If the growth receptor gene correctly enters cells, it will start expressing the receptor.

In a minority of cases, gene therapy has been associated with excessive growth of lymphocytes: leukaemia.

**Fig. 3.48.3** Gene therapy for X-linked SCID.

# 49. HIV: immunological features

## Questions
- Describe the life cycle of HIV.
- What are the key immunological responses to HIV and why do they fail?
- What are the three phases of HIV infection?
- What do viral load and CD4 counts measure?

## RETROVIRUSES

Retroviruses have small RNA genomes that contain just three major genes: for its envelope, reverse transcriptase and protease. HIV uses its envelope to bind onto CD4 and chemokine receptors of T cells and dendritic cells. It then uses reverse transcriptase to produce a DNA copy of its genome, which is inserted into the host genome. Reverse transcriptase is an unreliable enzyme and introduces mutations into the HIV genome. This means HIV is constantly able to change the amino acid sequences of its three major proteins. This happens in infected individuals (who may contain many subtly different viruses) and around the world (where there are several quite distinct HIV strains).

## PATHOGENESIS OF HIV INFECTION

Using its envelope protein, HIV binds onto both CD4 and a chemokine receptor in order to infect cells (Fig. 3.49.1). These are expressed at the highest level on helper T cells, but they are also present on the surface of macrophages and dendritic cells. HIV infects these cells after it enters the body through a break in the barriers: vaginal or anal sex, contaminated needles or blood products. HIV can also infect the fetus during labour or babies via breast milk. Sexual transmission is the most important route of spread, during which HIV infects mucosal dendritic cells and macrophages. These cells migrate to the lymph nodes and infect helper T cells.

HIV may lie dormant in cells for many years and only produces new viral RNA from DNA if the host cell is activated, for example by antigen. HIV does not necessarily damage infected cells, although they may not function normally. If an infected cell is activated, viral transcription takes place and infection spreads to other cells. High levels of viral transcription can kill infected cells.

## IMMUNE RESPONSES TO HIV

As is the case for many viruses (see, for example, influenza, Chapter 25), antibodies can provide a degree of protection in the

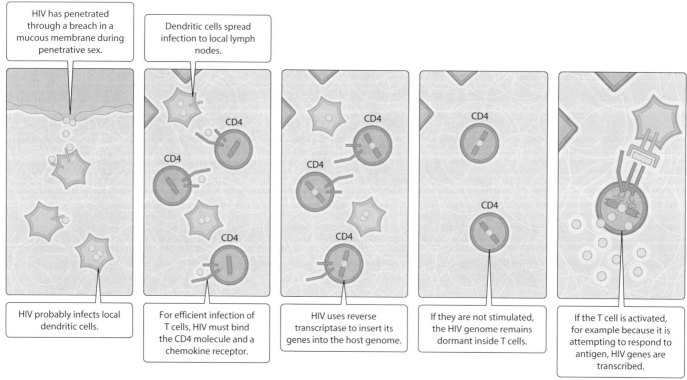

**Fig. 3.49.1** Infection by HIV.

very early phases of infection. However, antibody-mediated protection is only partially effective for HIV. Cytotoxic T cells are a much more important defence. In a very small minority of exposed but uninfected people, cytotoxic T cells can produce sterilizing immunity against HIV.

In most cases, cytotoxic T cells are not able to sustain a response against established HIV infection for very long. This is in part because cytotoxic T cells are not receiving adequate Th1 help, because Th1 cells have been destroyed. In addition, HIV mutates and escapes from any cytotoxic response that develops. The result is that HIV is gradually able to evade any immune response made against it.

## NATURAL HISTORY

During the first few weeks of HIV infection there is very active viral replication. This is brought under control by the response from cytotoxic T cells. Some individuals develop symptoms such as a fever or a rash during **HIV seroconversion illness**, so called because patients convert from being HIV antibody negative to positive at this time. This phase is followed by a long phase with no symptoms, which may last years. Even though the patient remains well during **asymptomatic infection**, HIV is actively replicating and T cells are gradually being destroyed.

The majority of patients eventually experience significant damage to the immune system. The patient will then develop opportunist infections, particularly with intracellular pathogens, which are diagnostic of the **acquired immunodeficiency syndrome** (**AIDS**). Patients with AIDS also develop malignancies, especially lymphoma and Kaposi sarcoma, driven by Epstein–Barr virus and human herpesvirus 8, respectively.

### MONITORING HIV INFECTION

Monitoring HIV infection is important in order to make decisions about therapy. During asymptomatic HIV infection, laboratory tests are required to show how much HIV is replicating. This is done by measuring plasma **viral load**—the amount of HIV RNA in the blood—and the blood **CD4 cell count**—a measure of the level of surviving helper T cells and thus an indication of immune status (Fig. 3.49.2).

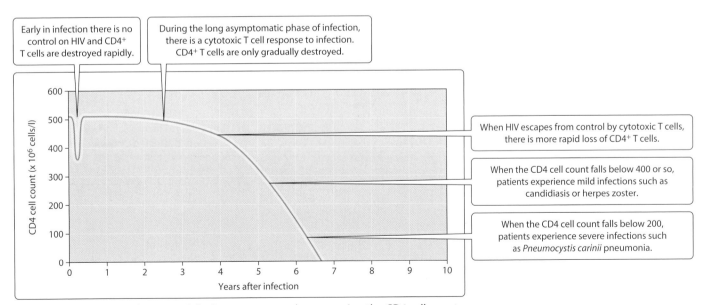

Early in infection there is no control on HIV and CD4+ T cells are destroyed rapidly.

During the long asymptomatic phase of infection, there is a cytotoxic T cell response to infection. CD4+ T cells are only gradually destroyed.

When HIV escapes from control by cytotoxic T cells, there is more rapid loss of CD4+ T cells.

When the CD4 cell count falls below 400 or so, patients experience mild infections such as candidiasis or herpes zoster.

When the CD4 cell count falls below 200, patients experience severe infections such as *Pneumocystis carinii* pneumonia.

**Fig. 3.49.2** Monitoring the state of the immune system by measuring the CD4 cell count.

# 50. HIV: what can be done to prevent and treat infection

## Questions
- Describe three factors that can affect the rate of HIV disease progression.
- Why has it been difficult to develop an HIV vaccine?
- What are the consequences of HIV mutation?
- What are the problems with antiretroviral therapy?

## ■ VARIATIONS IN THE NATURAL HISTORY OF HIV

Although most people who are infected with HIV eventually develop AIDS, there is some variability in how fast this happens (Fig. 3.50.1). Understanding what factors affect the speed of disease progression may help us to develop more successful vaccines and treatments.

HIV constantly mutates and some strains have acquired defects in minor genes that regulate replication. People infected with these viruses tend to progress to AIDS slowly. These HIV strains may eventually be useful in naturally attenuated vaccines.

Host factors can also affect the natural history of HIV. For example, HIV binds to chemokine receptors before entering cells. Chemokine receptors are polymorphic. One polymorphism, called CCR5Δ32, is associated with both a lower risk of becoming sexually infected in the first place and slower progression to AIDS if infection does take place.

The HLA haplotypes an individual inherits can also affect the rate of disease progression. HLA class I is required for presentation of peptide antigen to cytotoxic T cells; if an individual is homozygous for all HLA class I alleles, they may be less able to present important HIV antigen than an individual who is heterozygous at all HLA class I alleles (Chapter 13).

## ■ HIV VACCINES

There are two main challenges to developing a successful HIV vaccine. Eliciting an antibody response by vaccinating with HIV peptides is relatively easy, but antibodies do not have a strong protective effect against HIV. The first challenge to developing a successful HIV vaccine is the need to induce a cytotoxic T cell response, based on what we know about sterilizing immunity outlined in the previous chapter. To elicit good cytotoxic T cell responses, the antigenic peptides need to be delivered into cells and to enter the antigen-presentation pathway. The best way of doing this is to use a live vaccine (see Chapter 45), which would be potentially very dangerous.

The second challenge is that there are already many different strains of HIV around the world and a successful vaccine would have to elicit responses against a very wide range of antigens.

## ■ MANAGEMENT OF HIV INFECTION

The first aim of the management of HIV infection is to inhibit HIV replication and so prevent immunodeficiency.

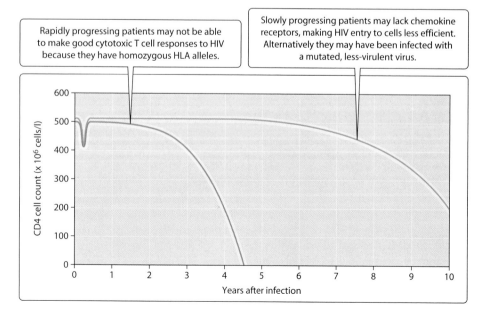

> Rapidly progressing patients may not be able to make good cytotoxic T cell responses to HIV because they have homozygous HLA alleles.

> Slowly progressing patients may lack chemokine receptors, making HIV entry to cells less efficient. Alternatively they may have been infected with a mutated, less-virulent virus.

**Fig. 3.50.1** The rate of progression of HIV infection is affected considerably by host and virus factors.

**Antiretroviral therapy** inhibits viral replication by preventing the action of HIV enzymes such as reverse transcriptase. Antiretroviral therapy does have side effects, and HIV becomes resistant because of its tendency to mutate. Because of these problems, antiretroviral therapy is not used until there is evidence of helper T cell depletion (based on the CD4 cell count) and on-going high-level HIV replication (based on the viral load). When therapy is used in this way, the CD4 cell count improves, potentially for many years (Fig. 3.50.2).

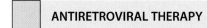

**ANTIRETROVIRAL THERAPY**

Antiretroviral drugs inhibit the actions of the three major HIV proteins: reverse transcriptase, protease and envelope. The biggest problem with these drugs is that if any viral replication continues while they are being used, resistant virus may emerge as a result of mutation. To reduce the risk of this happening, two or more drugs are given in combination. The viral load is carefully monitored and, if there is evidence of a resistant virus emerging, drugs of a different type are used.

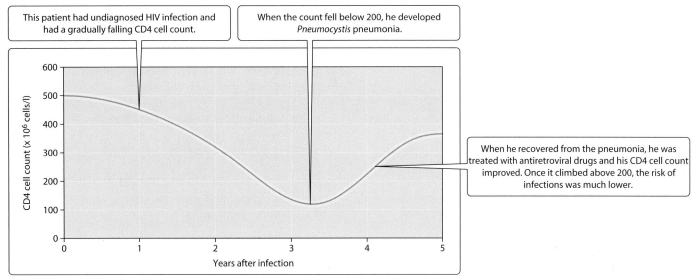

**Fig. 3.50.2** Symptoms experienced by patients, the CD4 cell count and viral load are all used to guide treatments in HIV infection. These include antiretroviral drugs and prophylactic antibiotics.

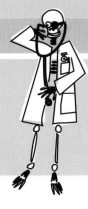

# Glossary

**Active immunity**
Active immunity is protective immunity that develops after exposure to infection or vaccination.

**Acute phase proteins**
Proteins produced at higher levels than normal during the response to infection; for example complement and C reactive protein.

**Acute phase response**
A systemic reaction to infection or inflammation, mediated by cytokine production, and characterized by fever and production of acute phase proteins.

**Adaptive immune system**
Part of the immune system in which genetic recombination is used to recognize specific molecules. Slow to respond but produces lasting memory.

**Affinity**
Strength of binding between antigen and antibody, or T or B cell receptor.

**Allele**
Normal genetic variants, occurring in more than 1% of the population. For example eye colour or different HLA types.

**Allergy**
Possession of IgE antibodies to a normally harmless environmental substance.

**Allogeneic**
Immune reactions to a genetically different member of the same species.

**Anergy**
State of dormancy induced by exposure to antigen in certain circumstances. For example, T cells become anergic during tolerance induction.

**Antibody**
Protein produced in response to, and capable of binding specifically with, a macromolecular antigen. Antibodies have an immunoglobulin structure.

**Antibody-dependent cellular cytotoxicity**
Process by which antibody-coated cells are recognized and killed by T cells or natural killer cells.

**Antigen**
Molecules specifically recognized by receptors of the adaptive immune system.

**Antigen-presenting cell**
Cells able to process antigen and present antigen to T cells on their cell surface.

**Antigen processing**
Digestion of pathogen-derived molecules into antigenic peptides, which are then bound to HLA molecules.

**Apoptosis**
Deliberate, programmed cell death.

**Atopy**
Genetic predisposition to allergy.

**Autoimmunity**
Recognition of normal components of the body by the adaptive immune system. Occurs in healthy individuals but can also cause auto immune disease.

**CD**
**C**luster of **d**ifferentiation molecules. These are cell surface molecules, each of which is expressed on different cell populations.

**Chemokines**
**Chemo**tactic cyto**kines**; attract cells to the site of infection.

**Chemotaxis**
Directed movement of cells, often to the site of infection.

**Class switching**
The process by which an individual B cell can, during maturation, switch immunoglobulin heavy chain usage, whilst retaining the same variable domain genes.

**Clone**
In immunology, a series of genetically identical lymphocytes, all derived from one B cell or T cell after receptor recombination.

**Complement**
Cascade of serum enzymes activated by the presence of pathogens.

**Cytokine**
Soluble molecules used to transmit messages from cell to cell. Interferons and chemokines are types of cytokine.

**Cytotoxic T cells**
Cells capable of recognizing and killing cells containing intracellular pathogens. Cytotoxic T cells express CD8 and recognize antigen presented by HLA class I.

**Danger signal**
Signals produced by the innate immune system to alert the adaptive immune system to the presence of pathogens.

**Granuloma**
A localized area of chronic inflammation, usually produced in response to a pathogen that is hard to clear.

**Hapten**
Small molecule, only capable of acting as antigen after combining with host proteins.

**Helper T cells**
T cells which recognize phagocytosed pathogens and stimulate the function of B cells or cytotoxic T cells. Helper T cells express CD4 and recognize antigen presented by HLA class II.

**HLA**
Human leukocyte antigens—also referred to as MHC. Genetically polymorphic proteins used to present antigen to T cells.

**Hypersensitivity**
Inflammation caused by an exaggerated response to an antigen. The immune response, rather than the antigen, causes disease.

**IL (generic)**
Interleukin (IL) is an old name for cytokine. The IL abbreviation is used as a naming system for cytokines.

**Immune complex**
Lattices of antibody and antigen formed in the body.

**Immunofluorescence**
Laboratory techniques used to show the presence of substance in a tissue (direct immunofluorescence) or antibody in the blood (indirect immunofluorescence).

**Immunoglobulin**
A soluble molecule composed of variable and non-variable domains, with antibody function.

**Immunoglobulin superfamily**
A family of molecules with domain structure similar to that of immunoglobulin. Each has a different role in the immune system. For example, immunoglobulin, T cell receptor and MHC molecules.

**Inflammation**
Defined clinically as the presence of redness, swelling and pain. Histologically, inflammation is defined as the presence of oedema and white cells in a tissue.

**Innate immune system**
The older part of the immune system which responds rapidly to infection, but with exactly the same response each time.

**Interferon**
A cytokine with antiviral effects.

**Lectin**
Proteins able to bind sugars.

**Ligand**
Molecule which specifically binds another molecule.

**Macrophage**
Macrophages are a type of long-lived phagocyte residing in the tissues.

**Mast cell**
Mast cells are resident in tissues and able to release granules during some types of infections.

**MHC**
Major histocompatibility complex. Gene cluster containing genes for cell surface proteins which present antigens to T cells. The human version of MHC is referred to as HLA.

**Monoclonal**
A population of B cells or T cells with identical immunoglobulin molecules or receptors. Monoclonal populations are often neoplastic.

**Negative selection**
The deletion of lymphocytes capable of recognizing and damaging normal host components.

**Neutralization**
Impairment of pathogen function by antibody.

**Neutrophil**
Neutrophils are short-lived phagocytes that migrate into tissue during inflammation.

**Opsonization**
Particles that have been opsonized become targets for phagocytosis.

**Passive immunity**
Transfer of effector components (for example immunoglobulin, T cells) from one individual to another.

**Pathogen**
Disease-causing organism.

**Pattern recognition molecules**
Molecules of the innate immune system capable of recognizing molecules characteristic of infection, for example double-stranded RNA and some sugars.

**Phagocyte**
Cells capable of engulfing and destroying particulate matter.

**Polyclonal**
A population of B cells or T cells producing a healthy mixture of immunoglobulin molecules or T cell receptors.

**Polymorphism**
Slight genetic differences between normal members of a population.

**Positive selection**
The ability of T cells to recognize self MHC with moderate affinity, and so survive in the thymus.

**Recombination**
Rearrangement of segments of genes for T cell receptors and immunoglobulin.

**Selectin**
Proteins which bind sugars on the surface of cells, for example to attract them selectively to specific tissues.

**Toll-like receptor**
A family of pattern-recognition molecules. Each Toll-like receptor recognizes different pathogen molecules.

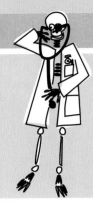

# Index